SIX STEPS
TO
SELF CARE

Learn the Steps of Self Care
to Reinstate Your Health

NICOLE CARTER, MED. CHES

BALBOA.
PRESS

A DIVISION OF HAY HOUSE

Balboa Press books may be ordered through booksellers or by contacting:

Balboa Press
A Division of Hay House
1663 Liberty Drive
Bloomington, IN 47403
www.balboapress.com
1 (877) 407-4847

Because of the dynamic nature of the Internet, any web addresses or links contained in this book may have changed since publication and may no longer be valid. The views expressed in this work are solely those of the author and do not necessarily reflect the views of the publisher, and the publisher hereby disclaims any responsibility for them.

The author of this book does not dispense medical advice or prescribe the use of any technique as a form of treatment for physical, emotional, or medical problems without the advice of a physician, either directly or indirectly. The intent of the author is only to offer information of a general nature to help you in your quest for emotional and spiritual well-being. In the event you use any of the information in this book for yourself, which is your constitutional right, the author and the publisher assume no responsibility for your actions.

Any people depicted in stock imagery provided by Thinkstock are models, and such images are being used for illustrative purposes only.
Certain stock imagery © Thinkstock.

Print information available on the last page.

ISBN: 978-1-5043-8327-1 (sc)
ISBN: 978-1-5043-8329-5 (hc)
ISBN: 978-1-5043-8328-8 (e)

Library of Congress Control Number: 2017910010

Balboa Press rev. date: 07/15/2017

CONTENTS

INTRODUCTION

From Sick and Tired to Strong and Happy

I wish I could say that I am just a naturally healthy person and that I grew up in a holistic minded family that raised me with all the habits I currently have. However, that is far from the truth. I was never a all that healthy as a kid and it took many years for me to find my path to health. In fact it has taken me 20 years to do that.

I grew up in Michigan, a beautiful state with plenty of nature to soak up. I lived in the city but had family farms, and grew a love for animals, growing food and tending land. My parents had divorced when I was 5 and I lived with my mother and siblings, a common theme of that time. I was the youngest in my family, but always loved to be involved in the cooking of food. My mom would go to work all day, and after school or on weekends I would often be cooking up recipes and concoctions for myself and family. I always had an affinity for nature and plants as well. I have a distinct memory of playing in the yard around age 7 with my mother lounging in her chair. I would pick different weeds and flowers, mash them in a bucket, add water and declare it my new magic "potion"! Little did I know how much this would match my skills and interest as an adult.

As a child I had frequent ear infections, for which I was given many antibiotics for. They were the treatment of choice at that time around 1980 and given out freely for just about any ailment, regardless of it being a bacteria or not. Recurrent ear infections seemed to be linked to my intake of dairy, after all my mom was raised on a farm and milk straight from the cow was not unheard of. The pediatrition recommened my mom take me off dairy and see what happened. To her amazement, the ear infections ceased! Any mother knows how stressful they can be, so she decided dairy would be out of my life for good. Around the same time, my stomach had become a problem though. I would often complain of stomach pain, and see the doctor only to come up empty handed. I was not drinking milk, and I was eating meat, vegetables, and grains. The building blocks of a healthy diet, or so we thought.

Fast forward to my high school years, where life was essentially the same. Chronic stomach and digestive issues was a part of life for me. I was also very tired and would come home and nap every day after school. I never knew this to be a problem, it was essential what I had known almost my whole life. Into college I worked hard waiting tables to put myself though college, and would frequently fall asleep studying. Again, normal and natural for my level of work and demands, right? I thought so too, until something amazing happened. When I was about 20 I was helping my dad to find a diet that would help him with his diabetes. He was seriously overweight and his doctor told him he needed to lose weight and eat less sugar. I thought I could help by finding a plan for him to follow and getting his food made for him. At the very least I might learn something for myself as well.

I had gotten into the college habits of eating junk food an drinking beer, and it was showing up on the scale. I was about 142 pounds, and was not very happy with my body. I thought that by helping my dad I would get some benefit as well, so I gave it a shot for the both of us and found a Diabetic Meal Plan.

Dad did not follow the plan, nor did he eat ANY of the food I had made him! I was discouraged for him, but I started on the plan myself, and stuck to it for about 6 weeks. Amazingly I lost 15 pounds in those 6 weeks! I had more energy than ever, the naps went away except for the occasional late night out, and I was motivated like never before!

Once I had dropped some weight and regained my energy, I began exercising more. I did fitness classes, aerobics, weight training and running. I even got my personal training certification through National Academy of Sports Medicine, and my journey down the career path of health and wellness was born. I worked as a fitness training for a few years while finishing up my bachelors degree in Psychology at the University of Nevada Las Vegas. One thing I learned while doing that was that MOST people I was training were women, and most of them needed to lose body fat. It was the rare occasion that I could train someone on weights and get them were they wanted to go. They needed a nutrition plan that would help them to shed fat so they could actually see the muscles they were building. So I started to incorporate the same diabetic diet I did for myself and my dad into my training. The success came as clients began dropping weight, even when they maintained the same fitness program. This was when I learned the critical role of food and diet as opposed to exercise alone. In the years that came next I would get more and more strict with my diet, taking out sugar, adding in more fruits and vegetables and event eventually taking out not just dairy but all animal products. I became full blow vegan and was somewhat extreme in my dietary habits. I would learn over the next few years some other critical pieces to the elusive health puzzle that would prove diet and exercise were STILL not enough.

The next avenue I pursued was herbal medicine. While working as a food server to put myself though college, I often had sore feet and throbbing legs at the end of every shift. I could not quit my job, it was my ticket to college and how I kept myself housed and fed, so I pressed on every single day taking every shift available. I remember being in tears at times due to the fatigue and exhaustion, especially with the pain in my legs and feet. Someone suggested an herb that I could take as a pill that might help with all this. It was called butchers broom and was supposed to help with circulation. I felt I had nothing to lose, so I went to the health food store and picked up a bottle. That night I went to work, took 2 capsules and started my shift. I was absolutely astonished. For the first time since I had been waiting tables, I went home with NO PAIN. My legs and feet felt completely fine. In fact, I felt energetic! I kept taking it and the results were the same every time. I was so amazed that I wondered how many other people must be suffering needlessly, and I decided I had to learn more. For the next 5 years I would study an online course that would ultimately earn my Master Herbalist Certificate, another huge milestone in my wellness career was underway!

I graduated with my BA in Psychology, was finishing up my Master Herbalist Certificate and decided that I had the time to pursue a more accepted degree in the health field. I entered graduate school in what was then called Health Promotion, now called Public Health. It was the most rewarding learning experience I had had to date. I learned so much about how people get sick, what kind of diseases prevail in the united states and how we can prevent them. During this time I learned that we as a nation did very little in the way of promoting health to prevent disease and that even as one of the most advanced countries in the world, we still had the highest rates of chronic disease. Here my attention would shift from one based on health and fitness, to one based on health and WELLNESS, a much broader way of looking at health.

There was a point in my life where I felt like my health was at its peak. I was about 27, I was a marathon runner, a vegan and heath and wellness advocate. I had not had kids yet, but was working on my Masters Degree in Health and had a lot of time to devote to taking care of myself. Fitness was still a big part of my health quest. I was not particularly lean, but fairly fit and extremely health conscious. I had begun to incorporate other forms of wellness into my life such as supplements, herbal medicines and teas to help me stay healthy and keep my energy levels up. I figured that as a vegan and someone who avoided all drugs, relied on plant medicine and had led a clean life that I was about as healthy as I could be. I would soon learn, however, that that lifestyle could only get me so far.

That same year, I was finishing my graduate exams when something unexpected happened. One morning I hit the floor in excruciating pain, and ended up having emergency surgery for an ectopic pregnancy. My fallopian tube had burst with an 8-week old fetus I never knew I had. I nearly died. It was a physically and mentally excruciating experience that also left its mark on my health in other ways. After the surgery and blood transfusions necessary with that kind of an event, I was on antibiotics, I was not eating well and I was depressed. I thought I would never have kids, and the idea of that was devastating.

To my surprise just a couple of months later I found out I was pregnant! I would take care of my body better than ever before, give it whatever it needed. I had the time to devote to it and so I read everything available regarding pregnancy, fed my body what it craved and napped every single day. I was a vegan, so when my body begged for meat I gave it, only because I had decided I would give myself whatever I felt I needed. I had meat and avocados every day, and gained myself a healthy 38lbs total. I had my son at home with my midwife and husband at my side, an amazing experience. All was well. Motherhood had arrived!

Becoming a parent was exhausting but rewarding. I tried to balance taking care of myself with the constant care of a baby, it was a real challenge. I managed to lose all my baby weight within a couple of months, returned to my vegan diet, started running and practicing yoga again. I was feeling pretty good. One thing I noticed however, was the ever present fatigue, which I chalked up to motherhood. It is a seriously demanding job. The struggle to get enough rest was always present, and fatigue was just a part of daily life. I pressed on, doing my best as a new mom, and repeated the entire process 3 years later with the birth of my daughter.

By now I had somewhat of a grasp on parenting (I thought) and had my routines set up. I was still battling fatigue, but at this point my energy was at an all time low. I remember a day when my daughter was playing on the slide, and I would close my eyes and rest my head on the slide, just for a few seconds as she slid down and went around to climb up again. I thought the exhaustion would never end. I could not understand where the fatigue was coming from, I was sleeping better than I had in a couple of years, followed a strict vegan diet, never ate junk food, went to bed early…It just didn't make sense. To make matters worse, I was getting sick all the time. A respiratory infection, the flu, a kidney infection, you name it, over and over. I was probably the sickest I had ever been, even though I looked healthy and fit. I should also mention that my hair was falling out, I was depressed and had no sex drive at all. I assumed, it was just the hard work of raising two kids.

I figured what I needed was a cleanse, maybe that would be just what I needed to restore my energy. I had already been practicing a raw food vegan diet for a year, how much better could I possibly get?? But I went for it, 3 days of juice and smoothies only. All raw, all fruits and veggies. This would definitely clean my body and restore my energy, maybe even make my hair stop falling out. Right?? …Wrong.

By the 3rd day on the fast I felt more tired than ever, was so depressed and moody I didn't want to be around anyone, and had a full blown yeast infection with UTI. Again! I had to admit that what I was doing wasn't working, so I went too see my doctor. This naturopathic doctor who did muscle testing and chiropractic sent me in for a blood panel to get more information. As he suspected, my hormones were all low, and my vitamin D levels almost non-existent. Added to that, I had rampant yeast in by body from the previous antibiotics followed by a high sugar and high carb diet. I had an overgrowth of *Candida Albicans* in my body, a yeast that can cause major problems when it gets out of control, and it was way out of control. I was the sickest healthy person he had seen in a while. He sat me down and told me that if I didn't change my diet, start eating more protein, that I would see more problems. Bigger problems. I had to get a handle on it. I wasn't ready to hear that, I was proud of my veganism and did not feel right about eating any animal. So I resisted his advice for several more months, still suffering from the same problems. I finally gave in and began with eggs. I gradually added fish and reduced some of the grains I was eating as a vegan. Things started to change, ever so slowly.

For the next several years I would transition from a high carb vegan diet to a lower carb high protein diet. My immune system began to recover, I was getting sick far less often, energy levels were returning and my mood and demeanor was improved overall. It took me a few years, but I had made some really big strides in my health.

A few years in, my dad had passed away suddenly and life was about to begin the roller coaster ride once again. However, this time it was stress induced as the death of my dad and also my 2 labradors retreivers, a major job change and relocation would take a massive toll on my health. Sometimes you can ignore health issues, people do it all the time. I ignored mine too. I had fatigue once again, regularly had stomach pain and discomfort, but it was the blood I saw that finally pushed me into action. It was time to get help.

I was diagnosed with ulcerative colitis, an autoimmune disorder that attacks the intestines causing inflammation, ulcerations, bleeding, pain, for several years. Overall, it's a pretty miserable condition. There are varying degrees of this disorder, and I do believe mine was not quite as extreme as some stories I have heard, nonetheless, it caused me much discomfort and many sleepless nights. When I was diagnosed with ulcerative colitis after a colonoscopy, I was told that there is no cure and that the only way to manage it is with a drug taken to control inflammation in the colon, sometimes steroids in worse cases. I was told not to change my diet because it had no effect on this disease, which is one of the most disheartening pieces of information you can receive. Being told that you will have a condition forever and that there is no cure is like a stab in the heart.

Knowing what I know about food and plants, however, I knew that this was not true! And since I am not one to take things lying down, I decided I would discover what else there is to know and find a way to beat this disease that often takes people's colons and sometimes even their lives. After much reading and research, I found that, although it is considered an autoimmune disease, the basis of the illness lies in inflammation (as most diseases do) and that, if I could find a way to take away the inflammation, then that was half the battle.

The other half of the battle was killing the fungus called *Candida Albicans* (yeast) that had grown in my intestines over the years and had never really been gotten control of. *Candida* is a fungus that lives in all of our bodies. When it gets out of balance (usually due to antibiotics and other medications), the natural flora of our intestines gets disrupted. This causes a multitude of health diseases and disorders, namely an overgrowth of yeast in the gut and intestines. When this happens, the body creates a lot of mucus (which you may never see) and this, in turn, causes inflammation in the body wherever the overgrowth is located, which, in this case, is in the intestines. Now you have a much diminished army of good bacteria to fight your illness, a whole lot of bad bacteria (fungus), and lots of inflammation...BOOM! The perfect recipe for inflammatory bowel disease (i.e. leaky gut syndrome, Chron's disease, and ulcerative colitis).

I will add to this that stress plays a major role on intestinal (and overall) health, and I did have signification stress at the onset of my disease including the death of my father, a divorce, plus major career and family changes. I have since taken an active role in managing stress through relaxation, yoga, counseling and meditation that have helped me tremendously.

Eating

I have an interesting past when it comes to food. I grew up eating a lot of meat and dairy products then went totally vegan at age 19, raw vegan at age 32, back to vegetarian at 34, back to eating fish and organic chicken at age 39, and now, as I write this, I am almost 42 and eat a healthy mix of vegetables and fish, organic poultry and buffalo. How many animal products I eat vary, depending on what my body is craving; I listen to my body. The only foods really avoid are processed foods, and I avoid sugar like the plague

I know many people that are passionate vegans yet are happy to eat French fries and vegan cakes every day. This does no favors for your health. The goal must be to serve our bodies so as to prevent disease, and one thing that will assuredly cause illness sooner or later is processed foods and sugar.

Other foods I avoid that many people will disagree with are legumes and grains. Both grains and legumes are difficult to digest and don't actually offer much in terms of nutrients, thus resulting in the gas and bloating that plague most people after eating them. The goal is always to get as much bang for your buck as possible, so to speak. The number one reason I avoid grains and legumes, though, is because they all feed fungus. I do eat peanut butter sometimes, but that does not give me any issues; even though many people worry about aflatoxins, I don't. I enjoy it, I buy it organic and I eat it in moderation mostly because I want to have less Omega 6 fats and more Omega 3's,

Since more than 80% of the population has an overgrowth of yeast and doesn't even know it, I think it's best to avoid grains and legumes for the most part. This will also help with obesity and diabetes, including extremely common diseases. I lost most of my body fat by ditching grains and grain-based products including wheat, rice, and corn. Most of these products are GMO foods, anyway, so best to avoid!

CHAPTER 1

Step 1: The Blood Sugar Effect, Eating to Balance Hormones and Mood

Let me just say, THIS IS NOT A DIET. This is a permanent change in your lifestyle and eating habits. Big difference! The way you eat affects your mood, energy levels, hormones, brain function, the level of inflammation you have, your risk of cancer, and more! This is why it's the first step in self-care.

This is a great place to start if losing weight is your goal. It's also important if you have a yeast overgrowth in your body (*Candida Albicans*), which you may recognize by fatigue, brain fog, sugar cravings, immune system weakness, yeast infections, or urinary tract infections to name a few. If you suffer from Type 2 diabetes, following a low glycemic diet is critical to reversal. Other conditions that will be impacted by this change include cancer, heart disease, auto-immune disorders, and inflammatory conditions, including IBDs, just to name a few.

It takes about 6 weeks to break old habits and begin forming new ones. So, stick to it, be patient, and wait for the amazing, life-changing effects to take place! Not all of these conditions will Be addressed immediately but in time you should see some positive changes in them.

Eat According to the Glycemic Index

Your body loves glucose. Because it is always available in your bloodstream, it's your body's first choice for fuel. When you eat sugar, or anything that breaks down the sugar in the body (such as a banana or a bagel) the blood sugar levels in your body rise. When blood sugar is elevated, insulin is produced by the pancreas to bring the blood sugar back down. Insulin is also a fat-storing hormones! This is what is happening in your body when you eat something high in sugar or carbs: your blood sugar spikes and you feel energetic, but later your blood sugar plummets and you feel exhausted, cranky, and hungry. This roller coaster situation continues all day, every day for most people, creating a continuous appetite, food cravings, fatigue, and mood swings. It is also very stressful on the body, so the body makes the stress hormone cortisol. Elevated cortisol can make you feel tired, hungry, lower your metabolism, and encourage belly fat where cortisol receptor sites are abundant. By eating low glycemic foods, we avoid the spikes and dips of blood sugar and begin to have normal hunger levels, decreased appetite, increased energy, and improved mood. Sounds great, right? Well there is more. You will also lose all the weight you need to lose following this plan, easily and without excessive hunger or food cravings.

How We Burn Fat

Since your body burns fat only *after* it burns glucose, the key to weight loss for most people is in reducing that glucose first so we can burn fat. By following a low glycemic index diet, you will reduce that glucose and train your body to use more body fat for fuel. We have thousands of calories of body fat energy at all times, so you will never find yourself running low on energy this way. Also, when we burn fat, the body produces ketones. This byproduct of the fat burning process is awesome fuel for the brain and gives you a heightened sense of mental focus and clarity. If you eat too much sugar and carbs, insulin levels will go up which encourages fat storage. When we follow this plan, we are more energetic and happier! Balancing the blood sugar is key to balancing hormones that affect mood, as well.

Avoid Foods High on the Glycemic Index:

Avoid any snacks made with any form of sugar and products with wheat and gluten. Most snack foods such as chips, pretzels, and crackers, sodas and bottled juices, candies or baked sweets are full of sweeteners and refined grains. You might be surprised to find that most fruits, root vegetables, all grains, and dairy products are also high glycemic foods that will spike blood sugar.

Load up on Foods Low on the Glycemic Index:

Focus on these non-starchy vegetables, proteins, and fats that won't spike blood sugar but will provide your body with loads of protein, vitamins, and minerals:

- Artichokes
- Artichoke hearts
- Asparagus
- Avocado
- Bamboo shoots
- Bean sprouts
- Broccoli
- Brussels sprouts
- Cauliflower
- Celery
- Cucumber
- Daikon
- Eggplant
- Endive

- Jicama
- Leeks
- Greens (collard, beet, kale, mustard, turnip)
- Mushrooms
- Okra
- Onions
- Pea pods
- Peppers
- Radish
- Seaweed
- Squash (spaghetti, green and yellow zucchini)
- Sugar snap peas
- Swiss chard
- Tomato
- Water chestnuts
- Watercress
- Cabbages (green, Bok Choy, Chinese)
- All Salad greens (chicory, endive, escarole, iceberg lettuce, romaine, spinach, arugula, radicchio, watercress)

Animal Proteins: (Food *quality* here is imperative, so spend the extra on your health!)

- Chicken (organic only)
- Fish (wild caught or sustainable farmed)
- Seafood (wild caught or sustainable farmed)
- Grass fed beef (smaller portion)
- Buffalo (smaller portion)
- Eggs (organic pasture raised)

Fats:

- Raw nuts
- Raw seeds
- Goat cheese
- Coconut oil (ok to heat)

- Olive oil, sesame oil (not heated)
- Avocado
- Almond, peanut or sunflower butter

Natural sweeteners (use these for baking, beverages, or any recipe that calls for sugar):

- Stevia
- Truvia
- Monk fruit powder
- Swerve

Condiments and miscellaneous:

- Sea Salt
- Black pepper
- Garlic powder
- Onion powder
- Pure dried herbs
- Mustard
- Sea tangle kelp noodles or yam calorie-free noodles

Also, feel free to enjoy coffee, green tea, and herbal hot teas (all unsweetened).

Eating Guidelines:

Here is how to do it! Look up glycemic index food charts on the internet. There are several, so just choose foods from the list that have a score of 20 OR LESS. Eat only non-starchy foods, no sugar, and stick to the meal plan.

Tips:

- Eat only foods 20 or below on the glycemic index
- Eat every 2 ½ to 3 hours, only small portions
- Eat until you are barely satisfied and never to full

- Do not eat from 7 pm to 7 am (or an adjusted 11-12 hour period) each night
- Drink 10, 8 oz. glasses of water daily, but more if you drink coffee and/or alcohol
- Eat as many raw, non-starchy vegetables as possible
- Avoid sugar, wheat, soy, dairy, and gluten
- Include the right kind of fat

Here are a few more tips to get you started. On the first day, write down your weight and, if possible, measure your waist at the navel with a measuring tape. Also, take a "before" photo. These are both great to look back at so that you can track your progress. Plan to prep meals as needed for each day. Being prepared will make a huge difference in your day-to-day life as people who plan ahead with their food are more likely to stick to it.

Sample meal plan:

Day 1
- 1 scrambled egg, 2 egg whites, and 1c. cooked spinach
- 1c. celery sticks with 2 tbsp. peanut butter or other nut butter (almond and sunflower are great)
- 4 oz. grilled chicken or fish with 1c. sliced cucumbers, 1 tomato chopped, and 1/4 c. avocado on a bed of salad greens with 1/4 c. salsa
- Chicken vegetable soup (homemade or low sodium) with green salad and oil-free dressing of choice with 1 tbsp. hempseed.

Day 2
- Power smoothie: ½ c. ice cubes or frozen coconut milk cubes, 1 c. chopped kale, 1 c. cup unsweetened almond or coconut milk, and 1 tbsp. ground chia seeds (blend well)
- 2 scrambled egg whites and 1 whole egg, 3 oz. ground turkey burger, and 1 c. cooked spinach or other greens

- 1 c. mixed salad greens with 4 oz. grilled chicken breast
- 1-2 c. chopped zucchini onions and mushroom stir fry, 5 oz. grilled or baked Mahi fish, and green salad with light dressing of choice

Day 3
- 1 whole egg plus ¼ c. egg whites with leftover cooked vegetables, such as asparagus
- Green veggie juice or milk shake (made with almond or cashew milk)
- 4 oz. grilled fish (or 1/2 can tuna) on bed of salad greens with light dressing
- 10 almonds, greens, or raw chopped vegetables
- Turkey burger (lean turkey breast, sautéed onions mushrooms, and bell peppers) on a lettuce bun

Day 4
- Breakfast salad: 1/4 c. oats rolled uncooked, 1/4 c. berries, 1/4 c. crushed almonds, 1 packet Truvia and cinnamon mixed with 1 c. unsweetened almond milk, plus coffee or tea
- 1 hardboiled egg and raw vegetables (choose above-ground vegetables only)
- 4 oz. grilled salmon with mixed stir-fry vegetables of choice, dark chocolate for dessert (about 1/2 oz.)
- Low-sodium turkey breast (all natural) with 1 tbsp. goat cheese and sprouts or micro greens
- 5 oz. grilled chicken with steamed broccoli and cauliflower plus small green salad if you like

Day 5
- ½ cup scrambled egg whites plus one yolk with salsa and cooked spinach
- 10 pistachio nuts and ¼ c. berries
- 6 pieces sushi (no rice) of choice, miso soup, Edamame beans (soy beans) and green tea

- 4 oz. turkey burger scramble and small green salad
- 2 grilled fish tacos with lettuce wraps plus fresh salsa and 1/4 c. avocado

Day 6
- Power smoothie: 1/2 banana, 1 c. chopped kale, 1 c. almond milk, and 1 tbsp. ground chia seed (blend well)
- 1 grilled chicken breast, steamed vegetables of choice, and 1 c. low-sodium soup
- Grilled fish or chicken topped with marinara sauce with choice of veggie side

Eat Fat to Manage Your Appetite and Balance Hormones

Somewhere along the way, it was decided that eating fat was a bad thing. Why fat was singled out is, I suppose, because it has more than double the calories of carbohydrates and protein (9 calories per gram vs. 4 calories for carbs and protein). While it is true that fat is more calorie dense, it also naturally occurs in smaller amounts. For example, fruits are often larger and nuts and seeds smaller, so we still eat fats, just not as much. For those people thinking that fats are something to eliminate from their diet, consider this: fat is a major source of energy and aids your body in absorbing vitamins. It's important for proper growth, development, and keeping you healthy. Fat makes food tasty and helps you feel full so you eat less! Also fats are an especially important source of calories and nutrients for infants and toddlers. Dietary fat plays a major role in your cholesterol levels, too. Cholesterol is important in manufacturing chemicals and hormones in the body, especially in the brain.

Essential Fatty Acids (EFAs):

Essential fatty acids (EFA) and omega-3 fatty acids are fats not manufactured by the body, so we need to include those in our diet.

They are needed for basic functions in the brain, and eating them can actually help you lose weight.

Omega-3 fatty acids come from plants and fish that eat plants. I like chia seeds the best, which is a complete protein and has many other health benefits. Omega-3 fats help your body create a hormone called leptin, which is responsible for telling your body when to stop eating, also, it helps the body covert fat to fuel. Omega-3 fats help you to feel full longer, balance blood sugar, reduce inflammation in the body, and help hair, skin, and nails stay strong and supple. Omega-6 and -9 fatty acids are also good, but the 3s are the ones we get the least and need the most!

Conjugated linoleic acid (CLA) is a potent nutrient, and the best possible sources of CLA are grass-fed beef and raw (unpasteurized) dairy products that come from grass-fed cattle. A host of research has been conducted on animal material, under microscopes, and with humans to determine the impact of CLA on disease. Results have shown CLA to be a potent ally for combating cancer (i.e. breast, colorectal, lung, skin, stomach), cardiovascular disease, high blood pressure, high cholesterol and triglycerides, osteoporosis, insulin resistance, inflammation, and food-induced allergic reactions.

Research on humans has shown that CLA has been beneficial in lowering body fat, with even greater improvement in those who combine exercise with dietary intake of CLA. In fact, research on animals has shown significant improvements seen in both reducing body fat and in increasing lean body mass. Previous studies have shown that CLA is said to reduce body fat while preserving muscle tissue and may also increase your metabolic rate

Since CLA cannot be manufactured in the human body, you must get it from your diet, and your best dietary source of CLA is grass-fed beef. The natural diet for ruminant animals, such as cattle, is grass. When left to feed on grass-only diets, CLA levels are three to five times more than those fed grain-based diets. Medium chain triglycerides (MTC) include coconut oil and palm kernel oil (non-hydrogenated). These fats increase the metabolism, help the body use fat for energy instead of storage (body fat), and curb the appetite since medium chain triglycerides are a form of fat that the body prefers to burn immediately rather than store. Unrefined coconut oil is a very large source of MCTs; on average, about 66% of it is MCT oil. This oil is great for cooking because it has a high smoking point and can be used in all forms of baking and cooking where oil is needed. In addition to helping with weight loss, coconut oil has been used to prevent heart disease, cancer, and diabetes as well as strengthen the immune system and improve skin and hair.

A Note on Fruit:

We all know that fruits and vegetables are good for our health. They contain vitamins, minerals, and antioxidants and have many protective health benefits. While eating fruit is often a better choice than boxed snacks or fast food, it might not be the best choice if you are trying to reduce your body fat. Yes, an apple is always a better choice than French fries, and it is obviously a great choice for travel or when options are limited.

Sugar, no matter the source, is a source of glucose. Many times, people eat large amounts of fruit, assuming they are doing a good thing for their body when in reality they are consuming a whole lot of sugar and preventing their body from burning fat. Yes, it's true they are getting a lot of other nutrients from fruit, as well as valuable antioxidants and fiber, but the reality is that, for rapid fat loss, sugars, including fruit, must be drastically reduced. Once you have reached your target weight, fruit can be reintroduced in small amounts.

With a high intake of fructose (unlike other dietary carbohydrates), your body can fail to stimulate the normal production of leptin. Leptin is a hormone involved in the long-term regulation of energy balance. It goes up when we get enough calories and energy and down when we don't, all to let us know it's either time to stop or start eating. The decrease in leptin production associated with chronic high fructose intake can have harmful effects on the regulation of food intake and body fat. In other words, with high-fructose corn syrup (HFCS), you never get those "I'm full" signals from the brain, so you keep eating even though you've gotten plenty of calories.

Our liver is the major site of fructose metabolism. In the liver, fructose can be converted to glucose derivatives and stored as liver glycogen. The liver can only use and store so much fructose as glycogen at one time while the remainder will be stored as fat!

The moral of this story is that fruit does have its benefits, so the best way of enjoying them without adding to your waistline is:

- 1-2 small servings a day
- Eaten early in the day
- Eaten all by themselves
- Whole forms only, *no juice!*

Should You Count Your Calories?

I never count calories because I am more focused on the kind of food I am eating. If I am eating the right foods, and listening to my body to know how much I need, there is no need to count calories. It is a very time consuming task that can also make you a bit neurotic to focus on every day. A calorie is a unit of heat burned within the muscle, and only muscle can burn fat. Carbohydrates and proteins are 4 calories per gram, and fat is 9 calories per gram; alcohol is 7. There are 3,500 calories in one pound of fat, so to lose 1 lb. per week, you will need to do the math:

250 calories less in calories each day (1 can of soda)
250 calories expended through movement each day
= 500 calorie deficit each day x 7 days = 3500 calories (1 lb.)

For this reason, even though fat is low glycemic, it is high in calories, so we still need to use moderation when eating it. You do want to eat fat because it helps you feel satiated and supports many functions in your body including hormone production.

Blood Sugar and Body Fat

When you expend energy though regular daily activity or exercise, your body uses up the first available fuel source: glucose. You build up glucose in your blood by eating carbohydrates (i.e. grains, legumes, fruit, vegetables). Until you have used up the glucose immediately available in your body, your body will not use fat for fuel! Reducing the amount of glucose to only what you really need helps you switch to actually using fat as fuel.

Glycemic Ratings

By choosing foods lower on the glycemic index rating, you are putting less glucose into your blood stream at any one given time. Eventually, everything will enter the blood stream; however, high glycemic foods "dump" sugar into the blood causing spikes and lows (cravings) and reducing the ability to tap into the body for energy. Choose foods that are higher on the glycemic index rating only before midday so you have longer to burn them off.

Typically the more sugar and starch the food has, the higher the glycemic rating will be. Proteins and non–starchy vegetables such as salad, green beans, tomatoes etc. are the lowest on the glycemic index. The purest form of sugar for your body is glucose, so it has a rating of 100, the highest. The goal is to eat foods lowest on glycemic rating so as not to dump glucose into the blood stream.

Meal Frequency

By eating 5-6 small, snack–size meals (about 250–300 calories each), your blood sugar stays balanced. Try to get protein, fat, and carbohydrates (vegetables) into each mini meal. Eating in this way also prevents binge eating as small meals help train your body to eat smaller portions.

Eating foods high in protein and low on the glycemic index will prevent spikes and dips in blood sugar while reducing hunger and food cravings that set you back.

We will be discussing your eating and fasting windows later, but, for now, just consider that they are 12 hours for each. At night, you will fast for at least 12 hours. During the day, your window for eating is also about 12 hours. As your blood sugar gets more balanced, it's best to extend that 12-hour fasting window wider and wider, until, eventually, you're up to 18 hours of fasting. This has multiple health benefits including faster weight loss, increased energy, improved detoxification, increased human grown hormone (HGH) production, and anti-aging effects on the body!

In the next few sections, I will be discussing some examples of foods and where they fall on the glycemic index. It is a good idea to become familiar with different foods so you understand how they all fit together.

Whole Wheat Is Not Healthy!

When we eat grains, no matter what they are, we fill our body with carbohydrates that turns into glucose in large amounts and "fill the glucose tank," so to speak. No matter the grain, this is what happens. Wheat is the most commonly consumed grain and is now one of the most common to also cause allergic reactions and other problems you may not even know are happening. It is also now almost entirely a GMO food, which is very dangerous for your body. Always avoid GMOs!

According to statistics from the University of Chicago Celiac Disease Center, an average of one out of every 133 otherwise healthy people in the United States suffers from the digestive disease known as celiac disease (CD), which is an intolerance to gluten.[1] Some of the symptoms associated with gluten intolerance include: digestive issues such as gas, bloating, diarrhea and even constipation; fatigue, brain fog, or feeling tired after eating a meal that contains gluten; diagnosis of an autoimmune disease; neurologic symptoms such as dizziness or a feeling of being off balance; hormone imbalances such as PMS, PCOS, or unexplained infertility; migraines; diagnosis of

---

[1] http://www.uchospitals.edu/specialties/celiac/

chronic fatigue or fibromyalgia; inflammation, swelling, or pain in your joints such as fingers, knees, or hips; and mood issues such as anxiety, depression, mood swings, and ADD.

What to Trash and What to Stock

For most people, the kitchen is where most of the eating happens. We typically eat whatever is there! By stocking only what you should be eating and keeping a few favorites on hand, you will avoid binging and straying off the eating plan.

Trash:

- Anything made with corn syrup
- Products with wheat, flour, or sugar (must read labels)
- Most snack foods such as chips, pretzels, and crackers
- Sodas and bottled juices
- Candy
- Boxed cereal

Stock:

- Drinks: sparkling water, non-caloric bottled teas (no sweeteners added), and raw apple cider vinegar.
- Snacks: raw almonds or other raw nuts, seaweed snacks, and protein powder that is low in sugar and free of chemicals (try Moon Juice, plant-based protein)
- Vegetables that keep well such as spaghetti squash and onions.
- Sweeteners: Stevia, Truvia, or Pyure, monk fruit powder, or swerve
- Miscellaneous green and herbal hot teas, Himalayan sea salt, garlic powder, and red wine vinegar

Cold Food Essentials:

Make sure there is always food ready like chopped vegetables, hard-boiled eggs, salsa for topping, and freshly washed salads.

- Milks: choose unsweetened almond milk or unsweetened coconut milk as these have the lowest glycemic rating and lots of nutrients Exchange all dairy products with non-dairy versions based on almond or coconut; you can always make your own!

- Eggs: eggs provide lots of protein and can be used several ways; I suggest keeping a few hard-boiled for a snack and plenty fresh ones around for your protein at meals especially if you don't eat meat, and I recommend that you choose pasture-raised eggs or organic eggs whenever possible and use the whole egg, unless you want many at one time, which is when you can use 1 whole egg and a few egg whites.

Ditch Dairy for a Lean Body, Flat Belly, and Better Health

American culture has adopted dairy as an essential part of a healthy diet. What we were not told though is that, after the age of 3, we lose the digestive enzyme to process dairy products. Furthermore, we are the only species on the planet that consumes another species' milk. Milk is not health food. It is not essential for the body, except as infants and in the form of mothers' milk.

We need calcium and vitamin D for our structural system, our immune system, and other essential functions; however, these are elements that are found in the earth, which plants contain by absorbing them through their roots. We can consume plants and obtain all the nutrients we need without consuming lactose from another animals. In addition, we know that too much protein contributes to osteoporosis because when the body becomes too acidic and calcium is pulled from the bones to lower the PH of the body toward alkaline, which in turn weakens the bones.

In fact, we consume more than double the recommended daily dosage of calcium yet have more incidences of osteoporosis than any other country. Dairy products have been linked as a cause of osteoporosis due to the fact that calcium added to milk may inhibit the vitamin D conversion into its active form. And on that note, Vitamin D is a hormone that is manufactured in the body (skin) with the help of sunlight. So, in theory, 90% of our Vitamin D comes from sunlight! Not Milk!

Aside from bones, there are other concerns about consuming dairy such as disease risk, toxins, allergic reactions, and body fat. Dairy is one of the many controversial issues about health, but evidence is continually surfacing that proves milk does not do a body good.

One last note on the dairy debacle has to do with probiotics. Yes, it is true your gut loves probiotics, which is the "good" bacteria that helps with digestion and immune function. Also, it's true that dairy loses most of its lactose when its fermented and turned into cultured yogurt. That being said, I think its fair to say dairy in the form of yogurt or kefir is far superior to milk and cheese; however, it's still not necessary for probiotic source or gut health. Probiotics are living organisms, and they, too, need to eat to survive. So wouldn't it make sense to feed the probiotic rather than just try consuming more? A pre-biotic is the actual fibers that help probiotics to flourish in the gut, so by consuming them in the form of plants, you naturally help establish the good bacteria. If that still seems not to be enough, probiotics are in just about all fermented foods. My favorite choices that do not involve dairy are Kombucha tea (made from a fermented mushroom culture) and unpasteurized sauerkraut (fermented cabbage). There are plenty of sources out there, all of them with their own benefits.

Why Goat Cheese is Healthier than Cow Cheese:

Goat cheese, like goat milk, is easier on the human digestive system and lower in calories, cholesterol, and fat than its bovine counterpart. In addition, cheese from goat's milk is a good source of calcium, protein, vitamin A, vitamin K, phosphorus, niacin, and thiamin. Dr. George Haenlein of the University of Delaware points out that the fats found in goat milk products are closest to human milk, which is easier for the body to process than those found in cow's milk.[2]

Goat cheese has a chemical profile that makes it favorable for people who suffer from aversions to dairy products made from cow's milk. Goat cheese contains less lactose than that from cows and contains smaller fat globules, which make the cheese easier to digest. A serving of goat cheese generally contains fewer harmful substances than a typical brand of cow's cheese, while providing similar, if not more, vitamin and mineral content.

A 1 oz. serving of a typical brand of goat cheese contains 70 calories, 45 of which are from fat. A 1 oz. serving of a typical brand of cheddar cheese, however, contains 110 calories and 80 from fat. If you substitute a serving of goat cheese for cheddar each day for a week, then you will cut nearly 300 calories from your diet.

The Detox Effect

Every living organism accumulates toxins in their body. They come in through food, drink, air, and from contact with the skin. Toxins circulate through the body in the blood and eventually make their way to your liver where they are then stored in body fat (what we are trying to get rid of).

When you stop feeding the body sugar, you will start shedding body fat and, as a result, releasing toxins that have been stored there for a long time. It's crucial to help the body rid them in as many ways as possible. Even though our bodies are designed to detoxify themselves, we are rarely able to keep up with the high toxic load we are faced with on a daily basis. Below are a few things you can do to help your body through the detoxification process.

---

[2]   Haeniein, George. "Lipids And Proteins In Milk, Particularly Goat Milk." *Lipids And Proteins In Milk, Particularly Goat Milk.* University of Delaware, n.d. Web. 03 June 2017.

- Dry Brushing: Using a large bristle brush, and without getting wet, scrub your entire body from feet to head in circular motions using the dry brush. This will exfoliate your skin, allowing the skin to breathe and detoxify itself. It also is great for increasing circulation.
- Hydrate: Try to drink 1 gallon of water with the juice of 3 lemons, ½ c. chopped ginger, and stevia to taste, if you like. This is great to flush the kidneys and helps to increase perspiration (ginger is a diaphoretic) while stimulating the production of bile in the liver.
- Love Your Liver: Utilize any foods or supplements that help to detoxify the liver. These include dandelion leaf (eat the greens or make tea), turmeric root (tea), beet greens, peppermint tea, and chicory root tea/coffee substitute. Use these liberally.
- Perspire: Use sweating therapy as was done among Native Americans for its cleansing attributes. The best ways are 20 minutes in a sauna, either a dry sauna or an infrared sauna. If you do not have access to any of these, then you can wear warm clothing and do mild activity to the extent that it promotes sweating. A hot yoga class is a great way to detox via sweating, as well. Be sure to drink salted water afterwards (1/2 tsp. Himalayan salt per 16 oz. water).
- Go #2: Take magnesium at night if you get constipated. You can also use herbs such as cascara sagrada, senna, and turkey rhubarb; however, those can be harsh and can cause stomach cramps. I recommend using aloe juice. I like Aloe Life brand, 1 oz. in the morning and at night. It can be diluted in water if necessary. Cabbage is also a great detoxifier, especially when fermented into sauerkraut.

Probiotics for Weight Loss and Gut Health

Every one of us is a walking ecosystem. We have our own chemistry and living organisms within. These organisms, called flora, can be both beneficial and detrimental, and it's up to us to help them determine their function. The good bacteria or "flora" helps with digestion and the immune system; these microorganisms perform a host of useful functions, such as training the immune system, preventing growth of harmful bacteria, and producing hormones to direct the host to store fats.

We can support good organisms with "food" that helps them to flourish. Foods that help promote these beneficial bacteria primarily include all vegetables that are low in sugar and high in fiber, but we can also deplete bad organisms through starvation and kill them off with antibiotics. Altering the number of gut bacteria, for example, by taking broad-spectrum antibiotics may affect a persons' health and ability to digest food. People may be prescribed antibiotics to cure bacterial illnesses or may unintentionally consume significant amounts of antibiotics inadvertently by eating the meat of animals to which these antibiotics were fed. In fact, 80% of all antimicrobial drugs sold nationally are used in animal agriculture.[3]

Alternatively, there are the "bad guys," or the detrimental flora. These guys feed off sugars and starches and are easier to cultivate and grow on these bad "foods." They love sugar! This type of bacteria is what is considered "yeast" and can cause many symptoms when they proliferate. Too much of them can cause candidiasis, or "yeast overgrowth," which can manifest into many different symptoms and diseases. The more sugar you feed them, the faster they grow and colonize in your belly, causing all sorts of havoc, like:

- A bloated abdomen and/or abdominal pain
- A slow and foggy mind
- A white coating on your tongue or inside your mouth
- Anal itching
- Chronic sinus problems
- Constant fatigue
- Feeling old and worn out
- Food cravings (especially for sugar) and food sensitivities

---

[3] http://modernfarmer.com/2015/09/cddep-report-antibiotic-resistance/

- Hair loss
- Headaches
- Heartburn, indigestion, and/or gas
- Intimate yeast infections and/or itchy skin rashes
- Mood swings or memory and concentration difficulties
- Premenstrual symptoms
- Red, itching eyes
- Sensitivity to molds, dampness, environmental pollution, cigarettes, and certain smells
- Skin fungus infections: recurrent ringworm, athlete's foot, (jock itch), or nail problems
- Sore muscles and joints
- Urinary tract infections
- Waking up tired
- Weight loss or gain

Although some of these symptoms may mimic other illness, they are often related to this imbalance in our "ecosystem." These symptoms can dramatically affect how you digest and metabolize food and how well you gain or lose weight.

The strategy for supporting a healthy gut flora or ecosystem is to avoid the use of antibiotics whenever possible; also, avoid eating sugars and starches that feed the bacteria and, instead, ingest pre-biotic fibers to support the good flora. Regular consumption of fermented foods such as sauerkraut (not pasteurized), yogurt, kefir, miso, tempeh, or fermented drinks also helps to establish and colonize your gut with amazing health benefits.

Food Addictions: A Common Disease with Deadly Implications

Since more than 70% of the American population is overweight, it stands to reason that there is an actual "cause" to this disease we call obesity. We know that it results from poor food choices, eating too much and exercising too little. We also know that many people have as much difficulty in losing weight as they do quitting smoking. What is often overlooked is that people struggle to control their eating and food choices despite their knowledge of its effects. For example, everyone knows that cheeseburgers and French fries are not healthy choices, and we know we should not be eating those nacho cheese corn chips, or at least not the whole bag! It is reasonable for us all to accept that ice cream, with all its fat and sugar, should be consumed in very small quantities and very infrequently, yet many people have no problem sitting down with a pint and finishing it in one go.

It's time to accept the fact that the foods we are choosing may be the problem. It might not actually be the fault of the eater, and it might not be that obese people simply have a lack of control when it comes to food! There is more evidence surfacing that supports the theory that food can be a serious addiction specifically with salty, fatty, and highly processed foods that result in obesity often. These foods are biologically addictive.

It's time to consult the scientific evidence on addiction as listed in the DSM-IV, the psychiatric bible and guide to mental disorders. One doctor, Dr. Mark Hyman, has demonstrated that the likeness between overeating and drug addiction is remarkable and clearly shows that food addiction is real. His research considers the following when determining whether or not addiction is present:

- Substance is taken in larger amount and for longer period than intended (a classic symptom in people who habitually overeat);
- Persistent desire or repeated unsuccessful attempts to quit (consider the repeated attempts at dieting so many people go through);
- Much time/activity is spent in obtaining, using, or recovering (those repeated attempts to lose weight take time);
- Important social, occasional, or recreational activities are given up or reduced (I see this in many patients who are overweight or obese);
- Use continues despite knowledge of adverse consequences (e.g. failure to fulfill role obligation, use when physically

hazardous) (anyone who is sick and overweight wants to lose weight, but without help, few are capable of making the dietary changes that would lead to this outcome);

- Tolerance (marked increase in amount and marked decrease in effect, in other words you have to keep eating more and more just to feel "normal" or not experience withdrawal);
- Characteristic withdrawal symptoms; substance taken to relieve withdrawal (many people undergo a "healing crisis" that has many of the same symptoms as withdrawal when removing certain foods from their diet). (http://drhyman. com/blog/2015/04/24/are-you-a-food-addict/)

Eating Low Glycemic When You're Working or Traveling

Finding time to eat healthy should not be a struggle. All it takes is a little planning and preparation. This is a program that you should be able to do forever, even while traveling and on vacations. Of course, it is ok to let the reins loose a bit sometimes, but you can still follow the plan and enjoy your food!

Tips for Traveling:

- Freeze items to get them through a full day of travel. (The best foods for this are whole or chicken and turkey breasts.)
- Snack-size cans of tuna fish and low sodium turkey jerky are a great traveling snack.
- Protein powders are pre-measured for easy mixing.
- Easy travel vegetables include green beans, pickling cucumbers, carrots, and dehydrated vegetables.

Supplements for That Support Wellness

In the quest to lose weight, consumers are always looking for the "miracle pill" to help out. There are literally thousands of products on the market, not necessarily because they work well, but because we buy them! In fact, Americans spend about $35 billion each year on weight loss supplements! The promise of a flatter belly and a toned behind lure us in to try just about anything without changing our diet or doing any exercise. The reality is, nothing replaces a healthy diet, and results are always compounded with exercise. Though some supplements may be helpful, of course others may not be, and some of them are downright dangerous! Here is what you need to know about what is on the market for weight loss.

Basic Supplements that almost Everyone Needs:

- A Basic Multivitamin: This ensures you get at least all of the basic vitamins and minerals recommended each day.
- Vitamin B Complex: Needed for energy production, nervous system, digestive system, concentration, memory, healthy hair, skin, and nails, prevention of cardiovascular disease, cancer prevention, and mental health.
- Vitamin D: Needed for calcium absorption, bone health, digestive health, immune health, mental health, anti-inflammatory, and cancer prevention.
- Magnesium: Improves sleep, relaxes the nervous system, helps to build muscle, and helps the body create ATP for energy. It also improves bone and teeth density, helps with hydration, relieves constipation, helps with chronic pain in the body, and helps the body produce enzymes. Suggested daily supplement is 300 mg at bedtime, slowly increasing to 500 mg. If you get loose stools, ten you can lessen the dosage.
- Probiotics: These may improve your immune system, protect and repair the digestive system, and keep gut flora in balance. You should get a wide range of bacteria strains in your supplement, and the higher the number, the better the supplement (such as 1 billion organisms), so long as the product is kept refrigerated.

- Antioxidant Formulas: These help prevent cellular damage, prevent cell mutation, help to prevent and reduce inflammatory conditions, and may prevent some cancers. Some great antioxidant formulas contain vitamin C, vitamin E, beta carotene, lycopene, lutein, anthocyanins, and flavonoids.
- Astazanthan: Astazanthan is a carotenoid pigment found in marine plants and animals and is often called "kind of carotenoids." It is considered one of the most powerful antioxidants found in nature, though it doesn't become a pro-oxidant in the body, so it never causes oxidation.
- Superoxide Dismutase: Created within the body, superoxide dismutase a powerful protector of cells. It breaks down superoxide, a damaging free radical, into a regular molecule and works to prevent wrinkles, rebuilds tissues, and reduces inflammation.
- Enzymes: All life processes, such as digestion and breathing, are regulated in part by a complex series of chemical reactions we refer to as metabolism, and enzymes are critical for proper metabolism function. The role of digestive enzymes is to break down the foods that we eat into smaller compounds that can be readily absorbed and put into the bloodstream. Plant foods naturally contain living enzymes; however, those die off in the cooking process. Try a plant-based digestive enzyme with each meal.

Supplements that Support Weight Loss:

- Seaweed: This gets a thumbs up because it is an ocean vegetable, completely edible, and without any stimulants or side effects. It contains naturally occurring iodine, which is great if you have a sluggish thyroid.
- Green Tea: Theanine in green tea helps suppress the appetite and increase metabolism. It does have caffeine in naturally occurring amounts in the plant, which is comparatively low when compared to coffee or "energy" drinks. There are no

known side effects or illnesses from consuming natural green tea or green tea extracts.

- Kidney Bean Extract: It is used as a starch blocker to prevent the breakdown of starchy carbohydrates into glucose, which is helpful for low-carb diets. White kidney bean extract can prevent alpha-amylase (an enzyme that occurs naturally in the body) from breaking down carbohydrates into glucose (sugar). By slowing up alpha-amylase activity, proponents suggest, white bean extract leaves behind less glucose for the body to turn into fat.

- CLA (Conjugated Linoleic Acid): Conjugated linoleic acid (CLA) is a fatty acid found naturally in dairy and beef, though it's also available in supplement form. Proponents claim that CLA can decrease fat while building muscle.

- Glucomannan: Glucomannan is a substance that is extracted from the root of the konjac (a plant native to Asia). It's rich in soluble fiber, which attracts water and turns to gel during digestion, suppressing the appetite and promoting the feeling of satiety.

Not-so-Good Weight Loss Supplements, so STAY AWAY:

- Hoodia: Hoodia is one of the better-known herbal supplements used as a natural appetite suppressant, but there haven't been any clinical trials involving humans as of yet. If you search online for hoodia, then you'll find hundreds of companies selling hoodia and cautioning you not to buy the competitor's useless hoodia pills. Counterfeit or fake hoodia is a real problem; it's been estimated that more than half of all hoodia products aren't actually the real thing

- Bitter Orange: After ephedra was taken off the market in 2004, bitter orange (*Citrus aurantium*) an herb similar to ephedra and has been marketed as a weight loss aid. Proponents claim that bitter orange can stimulate the fat-burning process, but bitter orange may raise blood pressure, increase heart rate, or cause abnormal heart rhythms.

- Gaurana: This is a powerful stimulant that contains high amounts of a naturally occurring caffeine-like chemical called guaranine, and large amounts can be dangerous, even fatal. (The fatal dosage has been estimated at 10 grams taken at once.) To compare, the average c. of coffee contains 65 to 130 milligrams of caffeine. Some very strong guarana-based supplements may contain as much as 350 milligrams. While this ratio suggests that it would take an enormous dose to cause death, even the supplemental amount is unhealthy, causing increased heart rate, jitters, insomnia, and anxiety. Also, this can damage the r adrenal glands, which is precisely what causes rebound weight gain.

- Undeclared Pharmaceuticals: The FDA released a report listing drugs found at prescription strength in several over-the-counter weight loss supplements. Some include Sibutramine, Fenproporex, Fluoxetine, Bumetanide, and others. Use extreme caution in purchasing weight loss suplements as this is proof that labeling loss can be sketchy!

- Meal Replacements: Meal replacements are often marketed as healthy food supplements with minimal calories providing all of your essential nutrients, but what they really are is a high-sugar, low-quality-protein milkshake. In essence, they are considered a complete meal because they contain all three macronutrients (fat, protein, and carbohydrate). Since they are in liquid form, it is easier to consume more calories in a short period of time since you simply chug down a shake while your stomach does not have ample time to signal your brain that it is full. This may lead to excess consumption. Since the shake is digested in minimal time, you will be hungry far sooner than if you consumed a solid food meal.

- HCG: A human hormone produced by the placenta during pregnancy, hCG is said to promote weight loss by suppressing appetite, increasing metabolism, and reducing body fat. HCG is the central ingredient in the hCG diet. It is administered by injection, but it is also available in dietary supplement form.

Injections come with risks such as blood clots and infections and need to be monitored by a physician. You can get your HCG injections online from overseas vendors, but you don't know what you're getting; very likely, it's illegal.

Balance your pH for Optimal Weight Loss

Blood pH, or the acid–base balance in your blood, plays a role in weight loss and determines how you burn fat. If the foods you eat upset this balance, then weight loss becomes difficult or impossible.

When our body pH becomes more and more acidic, it starts to set up defense mechanisms to keep the damaging acid from entering our vital organs. It is a lot of hard work for our body to neutralize and detoxify these acids before they can act as poisons in and around the cells, ultimately changing the environment of each cell.

To maintain balance, your body first tries to neutralize and excrete excess acid via urine. The body has a way of dealing with the excess acid by drawing calcium from the bones as a buffer to the body. In fact, an acidic body could potential lead to or exacerbate osteoporosis.

Signs of an Over-Acidic Body:

Obesity

Acid is stored in fat cells, and when the body becomes overly acidic, it produces excess fat cells to protect itself from the damage caused by acidity. The body then transports the acidic fat cells away from vital organs and stores them in cell deposits in other parts of the body. This not only protects your vital organs from failing but also contributes to excessive weight gain in the long run.

Joint Pain

Joint pain is another sign that your body may be overly acidic. When acid builds up in the body, the amount of alkalizing elements needed to neutralize the toxic acid increases, as well. When we don't consume enough alkalizing foods, acid remains in the body and gets deposited around our joints, causing pain and the symptoms of arthritis.

Chronic Fatigue

The chronic fatigue that many acidosis sufferers experience is a result of the acid's effect on oxygen levels in our body. In overly acidic bodies, oxygen levels tend to drop, and this usually leaves us feeling lethargic, tired, and restless. Not only is this condition uncomfortable, but it also allows dangerous fungus, parasites, bacteria, and viruses to grow more easily in our bodies because our natural defenses are down.

Allergies

When our bodies are overly acidic, our susceptibility to allergens tends to increase. If you are someone who already suffers from allergies under normal conditions, then you may notice that your allergies get worse when your pH balance is acidic. An acidic, oxygen-deprived environment produces more toxins and allows your body to absorb undigested proteins that lead to allergies. Moreover, a weakened digestive system makes you more susceptible to common food allergies.

Osteoporosis

Many people assume that drinking lots of dairy products and increasing their calcium intake will reduce their risk of osteoporosis; however, the disease is, in fact, less common in countries that consume less lactose. Some sources say osteoporosis has more to do with pH balance. When your body is overly acidic, it takes calcium from your bones, teeth, and tissues in order to protect you from serious problems like heart attacks, strokes, and cancer. This leaves the bones brittle and weak, making them susceptible to osteoporosis. The key to avoiding osteoporosis may be to keep a balanced, alkaline diet.

Continually choosing foods that produce acid can overload this buffering process. In addition, the acid your body cannot neutralize or excrete becomes stored in body fluids and fat cells. Once inside your cells, acid waste disables enzyme reactions, changes the process of metabolism, and stops weight loss.

When we don't get enough alkaline foods to buffer the acidic foods, our body will defend itself against the acid using the fat cells to absorb it, cholesterol will protect the arteries from being burned or nicked from acid or acid crystals, and even our organs will form cholesterol stones. So in theory, if our fat cells are absorbing excess acid and toxins in the body in an effort to protect our organs, then it makes sense that, as we move into pH balance through hydration and cellular nutrition, our fat cells will shrink by releasing the toxins/ acid.

Instead of focusing on removing all acidic foods, it might be easier to focus on increasing alkaline foods, which is more the issue for most people. In general, most people are not getting close to the recommended 8-10 servings of fruits and vegetables every day. By doing or exceeding this, we should automatically eat less of everything else.

How do we balance pH? By choosing foods that are alkaline to help the body maintain a blood pH of between 7.35 and 7.45. Any food that has a pH balance of 7 or higher is considered an alkaline food.

You can avoid becoming too acidic and prevent inhibiting weight loss by following a diet that consists of 35% acid-forming foods and 65% alkaline-forming foods. In general, this means increasing your intake of fresh fruits, vegetables, and nuts and decreasing your intake of grains, meats, and refined sugar.

Alkaline foods include all vegetables and grains such as millet, lentils, and wheat grass, and alkaline proteins include tofu, chestnuts, almonds, and whey. Some alkaline vegetables include pumpkins, dandelion root, mushrooms, eggplant, beets, celery, cucumber, kale, onions, peas, and many others. Fruits include apples, bananas, berries, figs, grapes, citrus fruits, peaches, and watermelon, and citrus fruits, surprisingly enough, add a high level of alkaline balance to the body. There are also spices that are considered alkaline, including cinnamon, chili powder, sea salt, mustard, miso, curry, and ginger.

Maintaining a Low Glycemic Diet

Once you get to a point where you are satisfied with your body, you can begin to eat foods up to 30 on the glycemic index. It's recommended that you stay there for 2 weeks and monitor your weight. If your weight goes up, then take the glycemic number back to 20 or 25. If you are stable, add foods up to 35-40 and stay at this level for 2 weeks. Continue this pattern until you get to the desired weight and are satisfied with your foods.

Tips for Maintaining Weight:

- Monitor weight loss regularly so that you learn what triggers weight gain.
- Create your own new meal plans from foods that are low on the glycemic index (under 20).
- Be mindful of the amount of macronutrients and calories (protein, fat, and carbohydrates) you take in, as these can also add on weight if not burned off.
- Be creative in your eating habits and try new foods and recipes weekly.
- Plan your meals with the hand Rule: 2 hands of vegetables, 1 hand of protein, 2 fingers of fat.

CHAPTER 2

Step 2: Inflammation and Gut Health

Inflammation can be your body's response to injury. When something threatens your body's structure (physical injury) or chemistry (allergy), the response is increased inflammation to protect itself. It can be acute (sudden and short lived) or chronic (long lasting). Such injury can also happen when the body cannot recognize its own tissue and creates an immune response or inflammation to protect against mistaken invaders. We call this an autoimmune disorder.

Inflammation can happen as a result of stress on the body, such as psychological stress as in money problems or marital stress. It can also be stress associated with physical demands on the body such as surgery or sickness. Stress on the body in the form of inadequate sleep can also trigger inflammation. All of these types of stress can affect your balance of stress hormone cortisol, which in turn affects your body's inflammatory response. This can show up anywhere in the body and in different ways. One example that is common is in skin disorders. Skin rashes, eczema and psoriasis are all inflammatory skin conditions. The intestines often get inflamed due to the foods we eat and the lack of good bacteria, so we see inflammatory bowel

41

diseases such as colitis, diverticulitis and Chron's disease. You may have inflammation in the body and not even know it. It is common enough to be part of your normal state for many people, and you just get accustomed to the way you feel every day.

Why Is Inflammation Dangerous?

Inflammation is actually a natural response by the body, and is not a bad thing when it happens on occasion. Unfortunately, most of us have continuous inflammation from poor food, stress, toxins, digestive flora imbalance, parasites or other continuous immune system reactors. Constantly being in an inflamed state is dangerous to your body because, once cells are inflamed, they can mutate into cancerous cells. Also, chronic inflammation can happen in the joints, skin, intestines, and other organs.

Chronic Inflammation and Autoimmune Disease

Is there a connection between chronic inflammation and the prevalence of autoimmune diseases? Some people think so, me being one of them. Much of the inflammation occurring from poor quality food or stress affects the gut, specifically the gut lining. Chronic inflammation that lands in the gut and intestines is particularly dangerous as it can disrupt overall gut health and be a major cause of Inflammatory Bowel Disease. According to the Mayo Clinic, inflammatory bowel disease (IBD) involves chronic inflammation of all or part of your digestive tract. IBD primarily includes ulcerative colitis and Crohn's disease. Both usually involve severe diarrhea, pain, fatigue and weight loss. IBD can be debilitating and sometimes leads to life-threatening complications. [4]The gut lining can weaken and become permeable, allowing microscopic particles to pass through the intestinal walls and into the bloodstream. This is referred to

---

[4]   Mayo Clinic. http://www.mayoclinic.org/diseases-conditions/inflammatory-bowel-disease/basics/definition/con-20034908

as leaky gut and has been suspect as a cause of many autoimmune disorders.

How Do We Reduce Inflammation?

For injuries, inflammation is natural for healing, but managing it with ice or anti-inflammatory plants can be very helpful. For chronic cases, such as autoimmune disease or allergies, there needs to be a whole-body approach, such as an elimination diet, detox program, or, especially, the inclusion of anti-inflammatory herbs and plant materials, especially the volatile oils (essential oils) from these plants. Some of the most powerful anti-inflammatory plants include curcumin, aloe vera, chamomile, and, my favorite, frankincense (Boswelia), all of which can be taken as supplements, used as oils, and otherwise applied topically to the body.

Foods for Inflammation

Anti-inflammatory fruits include: papaya, pineapple, Goji berries, cranberries, berries, cherries, apples, kiwi, lemons, and avocados. For vegetables: cabbages, broccoli, cauliflower, kale, ginger root, onions, sweet potatoes, spinach, beetroot, bell peppers, and mushrooms. Proteins are included, too, primarily as cold-water fish like cod, salmon, herring, and halibut.

Herbs for Inflammation:

- Turmeric: As one of the most commonly used herbs in Ayurveda tradition, this herb is a medicine cabinet all by itself. One of its main uses is to inhibit inflammation from occurring, but it is also a natural pain reliever (analgesic), which makes it excellent for injuries, joint and back pain. Use 2 capsules 2 times per day or as directed on the product package. Golden Milk (recipe below) can be used daily.
- Willow Bark: This herb contains salicylic acid, which relieves pain and reduces inflammation. It also reduces fevers. This

is the original aspirin; however, aspirin no longer contains white willow bark. It is not recommended during pregnancy and with blood thinning medication or for anyone allergic to aspirin. Use 1-3 capsules per day or 30 drops of the tincture 2-3 times per day.

- Ginger: This amazing root helps with inflammation by inhibiting prostaglandin production, and it is also helpful for pain due to inflammation or injury. It can be applied topically by placing cold tea bags on inflamed joints, which is called a compress. Use 1-3 capsules per day or tea bags as needed.

- Cayenne Pepper: This hot spice improves circulation and helps with pain when applied topically. Its capsaicin content can help with sore joints, sprains, and bruises. Use caution on sensitive skin! Take 1-3 capsules with food daily or use topically as directed.

- Garlic: Garlic contains the enzymes that generate inflammatory prostaglandins and thromboxanes, which help reduce inflammation. Garlic also contains allicin, which is an antioxidant that helps with inflammation. Take 2 capsules a day or 1 whole clove daily.

- Boswellia: This is also known as frankincense in its essential oil form. Boswelia is usually taken as a tablet or capsule as it is in its whole form. It is an excellent anti-inflammatory and helps to shrink inflamed tissue and relieve pain. Boswelia is commonly used for arthritis, asthma, and colitis and to help heal wounds. Use as directed.

Essential Oils Helpful for Inflammation:

- Chamomile: anti-inflammatory and pain relieving
- Marjoram: mild sedative and anti-inflammatory
- Eucalyptus: good for respiratory inflammation
- Peppermint: digestive inflammation
- Rosemary: join pain and vascular headaches
- Thyme: overall anti-inflammatory

- Clary Sage: best for PMS-related inflammation or muscle spasms
- Frankincense: strongest anti-inflammatory and pain reliever
- Black Pepper: overall anti-inflammatory

Recipes

Ginger Tea Packs:

Simply soak several bags of ginger tea in a bowl of water in the refrigerator, barely covering the bags. Take one out and drain excess water from the bag, then apply to areas that are painful or inflamed. Cover with a dry cloth to prevent dripping.

Golden Milk:

- 1 c. coconut or almond milk
- 1/2 c. water
- 1 tsp. turmeric powder
- 1 tsp. coconut oil
- 1 drop black pepper essential oil or 1 tsp. black pepper
- Stevia or honey to taste

Heat water on low heat, add turmeric and whisk blending well. Then add the milk and remaining ingredients. This can be consumed twice a day for relief or joint pain.

CHAPTER 3

Step 3: Stress Care for Adrenals and Fatigue

There are so many more things to staying healthy than just diet, even though it seems we spend so much effort on that one issue. The body responds to stress, as well, and it's usually in a negative way. This must be addressed if you want to stay healthy, and for those with autoimmune disorders, it's almost always a trigger for a flare up. Stress is related to several diseases including obesity, diabetes, heart disease, asthma, and depression, just to name a few. The day to day can show up as less of a chronic disease and more of a generalized fatigue with poor health, and this is usually related to adrenal fatigue.

Stress Causes Adrenal Fatigue

One of the biggest factors in your wellness experience is how much stress is in your life and, subsequently, how you handle it. Stress can be from the daily grind, relationships and life stressors, physical stress on the body, and other environmental stress. All of these things raise cortisol levels, and consistently elevated cortisol wreaks havoc. Cortisol is a stress hormone that is always present, but when our bodies and minds are under too much stress, we create more of it, which can lead to inflammation, weight gain, and adrenal fatigue. The typical scenario is feeling tired, which we remedy with caffeine. This might help for a couple of hours, but after that, it makes us feel more fatigued than we were in the first place. This is because consistently elevated cortisol levels (too much stress) along with not enough rest, poor quality food, and too much caffeine lead to adrenal fatigue. This is more than feeling a little tired for staying up late; this is a constant fatigue that persists day in and out.

To determine whether you might have adrenal fatigue, you might consider a saliva or blood test of your cortisol levels. You could also ask yourself a few questions, such as:

- Are you often tired for no reason?
- Are you having trouble getting up in the morning even after you've had a full night sleep?
- Do you need coffee or soda to keep you going all day?
- Do you feel rundown and stressed out all the time?
- Do you have a hard time keeping up with life's demands?
- Do you crave salty or sweet foods?
- Do you have a decreased sex drive?

Adrenal glands are responsible for regulating hormones such as DHEA, progesterone, estrogen, testosterone, and cortisol. When the adrenal glands are not functioning well due to overstimulation, the rest of the body is disrupted by hormone imbalances.

Adrenals suffer when they are forced to produce epinephrine (fight or flight) as well as cortisol, the stress hormone. When we live on caffeine, little sleep, poor quality food, and have too much stress we set up the perfect environment to wear out the adrenals. You can get your DHEA and cortisol levels tested with a saliva test; however, it's not a bad idea to use the suggestions below to address the symptoms. If after a couple of weeks you're still feeling exhausted, though, you should see your doctor.

Tips for Adrenal Health:

First and foremost, rest. Your adrenals need rest more than anything to repair. As you rest, cortisol is at its lowest. This is the stress hormone we are trying to manage, so getting 7 or more hours of sleep each night makes a world of difference.

Manage stress. Stress is one of the contributing factors to elevated cortisol and the norepinephrine that strain the adrenals. Reducing workload, working through personal issues, relaxation, meditation, and anything else that helps you manage stress are good for adrenal repair and prevention.

Eat for adrenal health. Your cortisol levels rise first thing in the morning, so eating a low-sugar, high-protein breakfast within 30 minutes helps keep cortisol levels low. Foods that are high in sugar or are highly processed should be avoided because they raise insulin levels, which also raises cortisol. Processed foods also lack nutrients the body and, especially, the adrenals need to stay healthy and prevent disease.

Eat herbs such as licorice root (if you don't have high blood pressure) eluthero root, maca root, rhodiola root, and ashwaganda root. All these have properties that nourish and strengthen the adrenal glands.

Essential oils can also help with adrenal fatigue. Lavender is known to reduce cortisol levels as well as chamomile and rose (proven to reduce anxiety in rats). Frankincense and lemon balm are also extremely beneficial for reducing the effects of stress on the body when used regularly.

Switch from Coffee to Green Tea

The natural products industry has latched onto recent reports of the latest and greatest chemical component that can help to safely and naturally boost brain function, reduce mental and physical stress, and improve cognition. The amino acid, L-theanine is prized for its mood-enhancing effects as well as for being very helpful in weight management.

Unlike coffee or caffeine or alone, theanine can help energize you during the day and help you sleep at night. If improved brain function and memory, improved weight loss, and a good mood aren't enough to entice you, then perhaps regenerating and protecting your liver is. The liver is the one organ responsible for essentially "cleaning" the body; everything is filtered here (and through the kidneys), so taking care of it is critical. L-theanine has a protective effect on the liver, especially against alcohol. It does this by increasing glutathione, considered to be the liver's antioxidant and detoxifier. Glutathione is destroyed by alcohol and chemotherapy, so restoring it is essential to the health of the liver and to the entire body. Theanine is one of the few ways to do this. It isn't hard to obtain, and the suggested dosage of 200 mgs daily can be obtained in a couple cups of green tea.

Meditation for Stress Reduction

As a yoga instructor, people assume I meditate daily. Actually, truth be told, it's very difficult for me to meditate. I have always had a very hard time quieting my mind and turning off the thoughts emerging from later in the day or week. Maybe you can relate to this. If this sounds like you as well, don't worry! You can still get all the benefits of meditation in bite-sized chunks. For busy and restless people like me, I recommend a 5-minute graduated meditation practice. Here is how you do it. For your first week, begin by setting a timer for 5 minutes. You can sit quietly or lie down, if that helps to calm you, or you can even turn on some instrumental music that is relaxing. For 5 minutes, just listen to your breath and notice the sensation of it coming in and out of your nose and lungs. Breathe in to the count of 5, and breathe out to the count of 5. Breathe in to the count of 5, and breathe out to the count of 6. Breathe in to the count of 5, and breathe out to the count of 7, continuing to lengthen the exhale to the count of 10. It's very difficult to think of the stressors of the morning or what's on your to do list while focusing on counting your breath. If you can do this easily, never mind counting and just strive for focusing on your breath. Once you have successfully completed 5 minutes, without your mind wandering, set the timer for 10 minutes. Slowly work your way up to 20 or 30 minutes a day. There is no rush, and even 5 minutes is very beneficial.

Essential Oils for Stress Reduction

The term aromatherapy was coined because of scent of essential oils is therapeutic. The scent of lavender is considered "relaxing" while peppermint is "invigorating" and citrus is "uplifting." These are true statements; however, we now know that it's not just that we like the scent but that it creates a beneficial chemical reaction in the brain. When an essential oil (natural plant oil from a flower or leaves) is inhaled through the nose, the olfactory system picks it up, and the limbic system in the brain is stimulated. This part of the hypothalamus affects our thoughts, emotions, the ability to focus, feeling alert versus sleepy or relaxed, and more. In this way, we can use essential oils both in the air as in aromatherapy as well as on our bodies to help reduce the effects of stress. We also know that lavender oil reduces cortisol levels in mice and could have the same effects on humans! Using essential oils is a safe and effective way to enhance your mood, relaxation, and even your meditation practice. Some of my favorite essential oils for relation and stress reduction are lavender, frankincense, wild orange, geranium, and vetiver. Try adding a couple of drops to a small bottle of water and use as a mist around the neck or the back of your neck during the day to reduce stress or to help you relax for meditation, or you might try a couple of drops on the bottoms of your feet.

Herbal Medicine for Stress Reduction

Plant medicine is just so great, and I always feel comforted by the fact that these plants are always there for us to use and benefit from. You can buy herbs in capsules, tablets, teas, and tinctures. Find the method that is easiest for you to take, and then choose the plant. Some taste better than others making them better suited for tea. Some of my favorites for drinking during the day include lemon balm, yerba maté, green tea, tulsi, and cacao. For evenings, choose a caffeine-free tea like chamomile, holy basil, rose, or even passionflower, though the latter one is strong and may cause drowsiness. If capsules or tinctures (liquid drops) are more your style, try rhodiola, maca root, or ashwaganda for stress. Check the package for instructions and dosage.

CBD Oil for Stress Reduction

Among all the other amazing healing plants out in nature is the hemp plant. Hemp is probably one of the most useful plants on the planet. It makes everything from rope to medicine, from food to fuel, clothing and so much more. The CBD oil that comes from the industrial hemp (*Cannabis sativa L.)* plant has almost nonexistent levels of THC (the component that has a mind altering affect) making it a very safe and effective supplement to help your body deal with the effects of stress and to help you feel more calm overall.

I think most of us recognize that we have a certain amount of stress in our lives. Many of us even recognize that we have it in excess, and we notice its physical effects on our bodies. If you step back and consider all you do in a day--all the work, the responsibilities, the computer work, the emails, the social media, the errands and family obligations, and even the workouts you do—the body is under huge daily demands. And, that is only the part *we* add onto ourselves. Let's not forget the demands placed on your body from environment such as toxins, EMFs and blue lights from devices, and other sources of negative energy.

Stress Makes Weight Loss Difficult

You may be working out 3, 4, even 5 days per week or more and still are not getting the results you want. You may be passing ice cream and choosing yogurt instead, or choosing pretzels instead of potato chips, or low-fat cookies instead of those Oreos. So, why then are you still in the same spot with your weight? Why are you working out and eating healthy and still not getting as lean as you would like? There is a reason, and it has to do with your blood sugar and your hormones.

Your body has been trained to use glucose for energy. We eat a banana or some oatmeal for breakfast, a sandwich with vegetables on it for lunch, yet we feel tired and still don't see those elusive "abs." The reason is simple; you have trained your body to use glucose for fuel instead of fat. So when glucose runs low, we get tired, cranky, and "hangry." To make matters worse, we are working out sometimes as much as 5-6 days a week yet still have extra fat around the belly, hips and thighs. *Why?* Because you are blocking fat-burning efforts with cortisol. You should not have to work out that hard! If you train your body to use fat for fuel, then you will not need to work out nearly as hard but will have the energy to if you want to!

There the problem with most "diets" is that you restrict your calories in hopes of losing weight with the calorie in/calorie out model. It does not work. You become tired in the afternoon and need caffeine to get through the day. You have strong food cravings, so you try to come up with crazy recipes to fulfill them, but it never works. Stop the uphill battle! True permanent fat loss comes from training your body to use fat for fuel, feeding your body enough fat and protein, restricting food at certain times to allow your body to rebalance hormones, and resting.

You see, it's a rat race in the gym, we go in nearly daily to burn calories and, we hope, fat. But all that happens is we burn glucose, and we fatigue our adrenals. And, alas, there is still no fat reduction. Exercising excessively could be burning up your adrenals and causing fatigue and hormone imbalance. What seems like healthy activity could be confusing your hormones by reducing cortisol so your hunger modulating hormones can do their job!

The Power of Sleep

Somewhere along the line, people have come under the impression that, the more we move, the more energy we expend, and the less we sleep, the more weight we lose. Enter boutique coffee and energy drinks consumed all day long! What we fail to realize during the quest for an amped-up day is that there are consequences for our not sleeping at night. Not only does excessive caffeine result in greater cortisol levels (which make us gain weight), but it also interrupts sleep patterns even hours later.

Sleep is critical for our natural body functions. It's a time for the body to reset, detoxify, rebuild, and generate new tissue and muscle fibers. Here are a few benefits of a good nights sleep:

Sleep May Help You Lose Weight:

Researchers have found that people who sleep less than 7 hours a night are more likely to be overweight or obese. It is thought that the lack of sleep impacts the balance of hormones in the body that affect appetite. The hormones ghrelin and leptin, important for the regulation of appetite, have been found to be disrupted by lack of sleep.

While doctors have long known that many hormones are affected by sleep, it wasn't until recently that appetite entered the picture. Doctors say that both leptin and ghrelin can influence our appetite, and studies show that the production of both may be influenced by how much or how little we sleep. This is often evident when a sleepless night is followed by a day when, no matter what you eat, you never feel full or satisfied.

Sleep May Prevent Cancer:

People working the late shift have a higher risk for breast and colon cancer, and researchers believe this link is caused by differing levels of melatonin in people who are exposed to light at night. Light exposure reduces the level of melatonin, a hormone that both makes us sleepy and is thought to protect against cancer. Melatonin appears to suppress the growth of tumors, so be sure that your bedroom is dark to help your body produce the melatonin it needs. It should be noted that getting enough sunlight during the day can not only set your circadium rhythms so you sleep better but also make more melatonin at night. According to the National Instiutes of Health, when people are exposed to sunlight or very bright artificial light in the morning, their nocturnal melatonin production occurs sooner, and they enter into sleep more easily at night.[5]

Sleep Reduces Stress:

When your body is sleep deficient, it goes into a state of stress. The body's functions are put on high alert, which causes an increase in blood pressure and a production of stress hormones. Higher blood pressure increases your risk for heart attacks and strokes. The stress hormones also, unfortunately, make it harder for you to sleep. Leaning relaxation techniques can counter the effects of stress, and there are also stress reduction techniques for sleep.

Sleep Reduces Inflammation:

The increase in stress hormones raises the level of inflammation in your body, also creating more risk for heart-related conditions as well as cancer and diabetes. Inflammation is thought to one of the causes of the deterioration of your body as you age.

Sleep Makes You More Alert:

Of course, a good night's sleep makes you feel energized and alert the next day. Being engaged and active not only feels great, it increases your chances for another good night's sleep. When you wake up feeling refreshed, use that energy to get out into the daylight, do active things, and be engaged in your world. You'll sleep better the next night and increase your daily energy level.

---

[5]   National Institutes of Health. https://www.ncbi.nlm.nih.gov/pmc/articles/ PMC2290997/

Sleep Bolsters Your Memory:

Researchers do not fully understand why we sleep and dream, but a process called memory consolidation occurs during sleep. While your body may be resting, your brain is busy processing your day, making connections between events, utilizing sensory input, and considering feelings and memories. Your dreams during deep sleep are an important time for your brain to make memories and links. Getting more quality sleep will help you remember and process things better.

Sleep Keeps Your Heart Healthy:

Heart attacks and strokes are more common during the early morning hours. This fact may be explained by the way sleep interacts with the blood vessels. Lack of sleep has been associated with worsening of blood pressure and cholesterol, all risk factors for heart disease and stroke. Your heart will be healthier if you get between 7 and 9 hours of sleep each night.

Sleep May Reduce Your Risk for Depression:

Sleep impacts many of the chemicals in your body, including serotonin. People with a deficiency in serotonin are more likely to suffer from depression. You can help prevent depression by making sure you are getting the right amount of sleep, which, again, is between 7 and 9 hours each night.

Sleep Helps the Body Make Repairs:

Sleep is a time for your body to repair damage caused by stress, ultraviolet rays, and other harmful exposures. Your cells produce more protein while you are sleeping, and these protein molecules form the building blocks for cells, allowing them to repair damage.

Herbs for the Nervous System and to Help With Sleep

Any herb that affects your nervous system has to the potential to help with anxiety, depression, sleep disturbances, and memory. If you suffer from severe depression, then check with your doctor and never stop taking anti-depressants without your doctor's knowledge.

- Ginkgo: This herb is widely known as a brain tonic and a neuro-protective (protects brain). It can help improve circulation and blood flow to the brain, and it also increases the synthesis of dopamine, norepinephrine, and other neurotransmitters. It can be used for Alzheimer's disease, dementia, depression, vertigo, memory loss, and poor vision.

- Valerian: Valerian is a natural sedative and helps you sleep without becoming addictive. It is used for stress, anxiety, and as a muscle relaxer. Also, it helps the body to increase its levels of GABA (gamma-aminobutyric acid), and it can be used for Attention Deficit Disorder as a way to calm the mind, for insomnia, migraines, shock, and stress. It is also a natural pain reliever.

- Passion Flower: This is another herb for calming stress and anxiety, and it's also an antidepressant, aphrodisiac, and sedative. Primarily, it is used for people with anger, hysteria, and hyperactivity. It can help you sleep, reduce pain, and assist with addictions such as alcoholism and tranquilizers. The tea can be used during the day and before bedtime to help with sleep. During the day, use only small amounts, such as 10 drops at a time to prevent sleepiness.

- St. John's Wort: This herb has been used for over 1,000 years to treat depression. It is also used for anorexia, anxiety, attention deficit disorder, fear, headaches, insomnia, irritability, and nervous habits like nail biting or hair pulling.

This herb can be used to heal nerves as well as treat nerve pain. It contains a component called hyperforin that helps to keep neurotransmitters in the body longer, assisting with emotional stability.

- Gotu Kola: Gotu kola is considered a "brain tonic" because it improves blood flow to the brain and supports mental function. Increasing circulation, boosting th immune system, reducing inflammation, and nourishing the endocrine system, this is safe to take in tea form daily. You can also take capsules as directed.

Recipes

Brainiac Tea

- 1 tsp. gotu kola
- 1 tsp. ginkgo tea
- 1 tsp. yerba maté tea (optional)
- Stevia to taste
- 1 quart glass jar
- 4 c. boiling water

Add herbs and water to jar and steep covered for 15 minutes, then strain and add ice and stevia. Enjoy the mind-expanding benefits. This tea got me through grad school!

Sleepy Time Tea

- 1/2 tsp. chamomile flowers, dried
- 1/2 tsp. passion flower herb, dried
- 1/2 tsp. rose petals, dried
- Stevia to taste

Blend all ingredients in a glass jar and cover with 2 c. boiling water. Strain and add stevia to taste. This is a great formula to make a large batch of, just brew it up each night or whenever you need it.

Note: Dried herb tea formulas last a year in a dark cupboard. Once brewed, drink within 1 day.

Herbs for Energy and Endurance: Adaptogens!

Herbs that improve energy and endurance are called "adaptogens" because they make us more adaptable to life stressors. Stress can be found in mental, physical, or physiological sources, and all have an effect on the body. Adaptogenic herbs help to prevent the stress from having negative effects as well as give us energy and endurance.

- Maca root: This root is from the Andes Mountains and works by supporting the adrenals. The adrenals affect hormone production and help us to feel energetic. Maca treats adrenal exhaustion from overwork, over stress, and too much caffeine consumption. It has the added benefit of lifting the libido of both men and women! Use 1–2 Tbsp. maca root powder per day in smoothies or other recipes.
- Rhodiola Root: It's traditionally used for its ability to increase energy levels for athletes and improve stamina and recovery time, and it is excellent for combating stress-induced fatigue. Rhodiola is one of the few herbs recognized as an "adaptogen" and was used by Russian Olympic athletes in the 1960s and by the space program in the 1970s. Since 1960, over 180 studies have been published on its chemistry.
- Eluthero Root: Eluthero root is another famous adaptogenic herb often used in TCM and Ayurveda. This herb assists mental functions, improves stamina, and energy. It's perfect for those who are sensitive to caffeine, work long hours under stressful conditions, and don't get enough rest.
- Ashwaganda: Popular in the Ayurvedic healing tradition, this is a pain relieving adaptogen herb that is used to mimic the action of the neurotransmitter GABA, which relaxes the body and helps to offset the effects of stress. It also increases the

availability of dopamine in the brain, lowers blood pressure, and relaxes muscles.

Recipes

Pre-Workout Energy Drink

This is a great drink to have before working out as it gives you energy, increases fat burning, and also helps protect your adrenals. Safe for daily consumption!

- 1 tbsp. dried eluthero root
- 1 tbsp. dried rhodiola root
- 1 tbsp. maca root powder
- 10 drops ashwagana tincture
- 1 green tea bag (optional)
- 1 glass quart-sized jar
- 4 c. boiled water
- Stevia to taste

Add eluthero root, rhodiola root, and green tea (if you want an extra boost of caffeine) to the glass jar and cover with hot water. Allow it to steep 20 minutes or more. Strain and add in maca, ashwaganda tincture, and ice, and sweeten with stevia if you like.

Libido Boosting Treats

- 1 c. raw walnuts
- 1/4 c. raw cacao powder
- 1/8 c. maca root powder
- 1 tsp. stevia powder
- 1 tsp. vanilla powder (or alcohol-free extract)
- 1/2 tsp. sea salt

Add all ingredients to a food processor and grind into a smooth paste. Using 2 tbsp. at a time, roll into balls and set on waxed paper. Chill in the refrigerator or store in the freezer. Use within 2 months if frozen and 1 week if refrigerated.

CHAPTER 4

Step 4: Holistic Detox for Fungus, Bacteria, and Parasites

First of all, don't be scared! We all have these toxins, and they do not leave your body in a 3 day juice cleanse! So, let's do it right with diet and our arsenal of plant medicine, and you must, of course, give it time.

Antibiotic Recover

We have finally started to pull back the reins when it comes to using antibiotics. For years, it was our first line of defense against any kind of bacteria and usually prescribed as a preventative measure. This may have seemed like a good idea 20 years ago, but today, we face 2 major challenges as a result of this approach. Those challenges are (1) antibiotic resistance and (2) digestive system disorders. We are currently in a state of antibiotic recovery. According to the Center for Disease Control and Prevention (CDC) antibiotic resistance is one of the world's most pressing public health problems.

Exposure:

In the United States, nearly every man, women, and child has been exposed to antibiotics via a prescribed medication from their doctors. They are supposed to be used only for serious bacterial infections; however, they are prescribed often at the first sign of even a minor topical injury when something such as iodine can still be used to kill most bacteria. We also have had years of doctors prescribing antibiotics as a preventative measure to a secondary infection in the case of viral infections, and the number of unnecessary antibiotics prescribed annually for viral infections is 20 million per year.

As most know, antibiotics are useless against viral infections as these infections live inside cells where antibiotics cannot penetrate. Antibiotics have saved many lives, no doubt, but due to overuse and misuse, we now are suffering the consequences.

Most of us in the United States have also been exposed to antibiotics via the food chain. A large proportion of antibiotics manufactured (estimated at 80%) are for animal agriculture. These antibiotics are given to animals to prevent disease, even though most of the diseases are now resistant to antibiotics. Still, animals receive them as part of their regular feed. This is then passed through their systems and can contaminate ground water as well as what remains in their bodies when consumed by humans.

Effects of Antibiotics:

Antibiotics have been one of the most effective medications every created; however, they also can create some of the most widespread damage, not only to our environment and the spawn of more resistant bacteria but also to our inner ecology. A common symptom while taking antibiotics is diarrhea.

Short-Term Side Effects:

As with any drug, antibiotics carry with them a host of possible side effects, which is what doctors are typically concerned with.

What can happen within a few days or weeks of taking them? Side effects vary with different antibiotics but collectively include the increased risk of musculoskeletal side effect, visual and renal systems, central nervous system damage, depression, hallucinations, psychotic reactions, and damage to the heart, liver, as well as the gastrointestinal system, which includes nausea, and diarrhea as well as hearing and blood sugar metabolism.

Long-Term Side Effects:

Candida is stored in the intestinal tract. Within 2 weeks of antibiotic use, normal healthy bacteria are killed off, making room for candida to flourish. While the short-term side effects are not all that common (except diarrhea which occurs in approximately 40% of cases), long-term side effects are less studied but appear to be more wide spread. One of the most common being the overgrowth of yeast in the body, bacteria called *Candida Albicans* that I mentioned in the beginning of the book, which is estimated to be present in as many as 80% of Americans.

The overgrowth of candida-causing candidiasis is not new, and the yeast was first described in the 1940s as a rare medical occurrence.; however, as antibiotic use increased, so did the incidence of candidiasis, and by the 1950s, there was an epidemic of yeast infections that matched the rise in antibiotic use. Illnesses associated with candidiasis include ache, sinusitis, athlete's foot, constipation, diarrhea, depression, ear infections, urinary tract infections, and chronic fatigue syndrome.

Another major issue common among adults is inflammatory bowel disease (IBD), which has been associated with prior antibiotic use. In an article written by Dr. Charles Bernstein MD, head of Gastroenterology at the IBD Clinical & Research Center at the University of Manitoba, he claims that it's not a cause-and-effect relationship, but it points to several papers published on IBD that suggest an association between antibiotic use and IBD.

Considering the prevalence and widespread use of antibiotics, there is a huge need now to rebalance the body and finally recover from their use. This requires healing the digestive system, killing the overgrowth of *Candida Albicans* (and subsequent infections caused by it), and, finally, reestablishing and recolonizing the natural antibodies that should be present within all of us.

Herbs for Bacteria in the Body (Antibiotic Alternatives):

- Olive Leaf: This unsuspecting herb is the leaf of the common olive tree that produces olives and olive oil. The leaves contain oleoropein, which dissolves the outer lining of pathogenic microbes, yet, it has no negative side effects for humans. Although it's not common to have any side effects, you should take it with food to prevent any stomach irritation just to be safe.

- Astragalus: One of the most widely prescribed herbs in Chinese Medicine, it is used to bolster the immune system and help the body become more resistant to invasive pathogens. It also inhibits viral replication, slowing down and preventing the spread of viral infections within the body. This makes it important to use it at the 1st sign of illness! This herb is very safe; however. it is not recommended during high fevers.

- Garlic: One of the oldest remedies for colds and the flu, raw garlic takes the cake and is always available. No wonder they call it the "King of Herbs!" It can help fight infections caused by staph, strep, and even salmonella, not to mention garlic is the perfect remedy for congestion and coughs as well as sore throats. Add it raw to your food, make soup and add fresh chopped garlic at the end, or even just crush a clove and spread it on toast with butter for a real "garlic bread" treat.

- Myrrh: This herb was mentioned in the bible along with frankincense and gold! It increases the motility of white blood cells that fight infection and is excellent for sore throats and tonsillitis. The easiest way to use this herb is in liquid drops, adding 30 drops to water or tea and letting it come into contact with the throat.

- Thyme: This simple garden plant packs a powerful punch! It has natural antibiotic properties as well as acts as an expectorant to help remove lung congestion. This makes a great tea when combined with peppermint to treat even the most persistent coughs. The best part is that it is safe with zero side effects. It's great for kids, too!
- Oregano Oil: This is extremely powerful oil, so be careful! It's used for stimulating the immune system, athlete's foot, candida, parasites, and warts.

Parasites

Having parasites will disable your gut from every truly healing! You must destroy and rid the body of parasites. Parasites can enter our bodies from our food, drink, and even our skin. Common sources of parasite infection include swimming in fresh water or streams, undercooked meats, raw fish, salads, and raw vegetables, but they may also come from food made in restaurants, poor hygiene, or from your pets.

Many times, a parasite can thrive in the human body and show no signs of its presence. Other times, a person will feel constantly ill, be on several medications (including antipsychotic drugs), and have no idea that a chronic parasitic infection is at the root of their problems.

Parasites Come in Many Shapes and Sizes

One of the most common parasites to infect human beings is a single-celled parasite called *Blastocystis hominis*. It causes abdominal cramping, bloating, gas, and, sometimes, anal itching.

Other Common Parasites:

- Tapeworms: They can grow as long as 60 feet while living in the human intestines, and there are currently more than 5,000 different species of tapeworm.

- Hookworms: If given the chance, they will suck blood from our intestinal walls.
- Giardia: Giardia is a single-celled parasite that is usually the result of drinking infected waters. It typically survives in chlorinated water and commonly lives in mountain streams, earning it the name, "backpacker's diarrhea." About 2.5 million cases are reported annually.
- Blood flukes: They mature first in snails and then complete their life cycle by burrowing through human skin and swimming through veins, but there are also other species of flukes found living in the liver, lungs, and pancreas. Blood flukes infect more than 200 million people.
- Pinworms: The most common roundworm in the United States is the pinworm. The most common sign of pinworm infestation is anal itching at night, which is when the female pinworm migrates to the perineum to lay her eggs. Children are the most common carriers.

Possible Symptoms Associated with Parasites:

- Chronic Digestive Issues: If you harbor a parasite, any work you may do to heal your gut will be constantly undermined. This is because parasites often create intestinal inflammation and destroy the intestinal lining of the gut.
- Various Forms of Mental Distress: This includes depression, anxiety, headaches, eye aches, and other vision problems.
- Depression, Anxiety and Mood Disorders: The gut is full of both neurons and neurotransmitters, specifically serotonin, and it makes up what is known as the enteric nervous system. The gut and the brain have a direct relationship, which is known as the "gut-brain axis".
- Autoimmune Disorders: The autoimmune flare-ups that have been documented to be specifically related to parasitic infection are gut- and joint-related, such as irritable bowel syndrome (IBS) and reactive arthritis.

Treating Parasites:

If you suspect parasites, you can work with a naturopathic doctor to get a stool test and confirm parasites. If you symptoms are mild or if you would like to take a preventative approach, Renew Life has an excellent parasite cleanse, or you could also make your own "bug bomb," as I will demonstrate in just a bit.

Herbs for Parasites:

- Wormwood
- Black walnut hulls (has been shown to kill a variety of parasites)
- Clove (the oil contains eugenol that is highly antimicrobial and can kill microscopic parasites and larvae)
- Garlic (this can be eaten raw or taken in capsules to expel parasites of all kinds)
- Papaya seeds (after eating the fruit, chew a teaspoon of the seeds, and this is best done daily)
- Pumpkin seeds (eating at least ½ c. of these seeds daily may help treat tapeworms)

"Bug Bomb:" Add 1 drop of clove oil, 1 drop of oregano oil, and, optionally, 1 drop of ginger oil to an empty capsule and take it immediately. You can do this every night at bedtime for 3 weeks, then take a week off.

Detox your Diet

One of the biggest ways we invite toxins into our bodies is through diet. This includes the foods we eat and the beverages we drink. The majority of people eat a significant amount of processed foods on a daily basis. Consider all the food you eat in one day. Is it all in wholefood form? Has any of it been processed and packaged? If not, you're doing well! But, if processed foods such as breads, crackers, cereals, snacks, and deserts are a part of your diet, then we have some work to do!

The main goal is to clean out all of the processed foods, food additives, artificial ingredients, and toxic foods from your diet. In addition, we should strive to add more green vegetables to our food so that we get more chlorophyll, which naturally detoxifies the body.

Another goal is to take a look at how our foods are grown and delivered. Buying *organic* foods helps to reduce the likelihood of eating pesticides, herbicides, and genetically engineered foods (GMOs), which pose serious health risks as they are designed with a killing agent right in the seed to keep pests from eating the crops; however, this doesn't go unnoticed when our body eats it! Watch out for GMOs; go organic to be safe.

One way to make things easier is to identify the ingredients to be reduced and eliminated as separate from the clean ones. Avoid anything that may pose as a toxin to your system, and utilize the clean list, which refers to all safe foods. This does not mean they are low calorie, low fat, or promote weight loss, though. It means only that they are not toxic. If it's high in sugar or fat, you should still practice moderation when having it.

Foods to Avoid

- Proteins: Processed lunch meats, cured meats, sausages, patties, burgers, fish sticks, meat analogs (Vegetarian "burgers or chicken"), standard eggs, egg substitutes are all proteins to avoid. Animal proteins are highly reduced for this program due to bioaccumulation, or the buildup of toxins higher along the food chain. If you choose to eat mean and animal products, then be sure to use wild caught fish and seafood (not farmed), organic pasture raised chicken, pasture raised eggs, and grass-fed beef or buffalo. Pork products are not recommended.
- Dairy Products: We are the only species to consume another animals' milk, and the truth is that we just are not meant to do that. Check the clean list for better options. Soy milk and soy-related products are not good options because they

can disrupt hormones and cause inflammation, the precursor to many disease. Soy products are also high glycemic foods that can spike insulin and are most likely to be genetically engineered.

- Grain Products: Enriched flours, wheat flour, corn flour, corn, soy and soy isolates are all in this category. These are difficult to digest and cause inflammation as well as skin and gut irritation in many people, and they also break down sugar and feed the *Candida Albicans* yeast.
- Sugar and Sweeteners: Corn syrups, fructose, glucose, invert sugar, brown sugar, maltose, dextrose, sucrose, Splenda, sucralose, and aspartame should all be avoided.
- Fats: Hydrogenated or fractionated oils, hydrogenated coconut (virgin is fine), palm or soybean oil, canola oil, corn oil and peanut oil fall in this area. Reduce oil consumption overall.
- Flavor Enhancers: This includes monosodium glutamate (MSG) and all artificial flavorings.
- Artificial Colors: None of these are safe!
- Preservatives: This includes disodium inosinate, pyrophosphate, nitrites, BHA, and BHT.
- Canned Foods/Plastic Bottles: These can be toxic because of the BPA (Bisphenol A) that can leach into foods. Buy foods bottled in glass jars, BPA-free aspic boxes, or frozen food.
- Miscellaneous: Propylene glycol, potassium benzoate and sodium benzoate, potassium sorbate, polysorbate 80, propyl gallate, and sodium chloride should all be avoided.

Foods to Focus on

- Proteins: Pasture-raised eggs, pure egg whites, hemp seeds, and raw nuts are all permissible. Buy organic!
- Non-Dairy: This includes goats' milk and cheese, nut milks and cheese, coconut milk, and coconut milk yogurt.

- Sweeteners: You can us raw honey, coconut sugar, coconut syrup, stevia, monk fruit powder, date sugar, and maple syrup.
- Fats: Good fats include almond, cashew, or sunflower seed butters and coconut oil, olive oil, sesame oil, ghee, organic grass fed butter, organically grown meats, avocados, raw nuts, and seeds.
- Baking: Healthy baking is made easy with natural flavorings and herbs, sea salt, and raw cacao powder.

Create Clean Menus and Plan or Prep Meals

Being prepared with the right foods means you won't skip to the packaged foods full of chemicals. Have food ready at all times! Start creating your own menus by incorporating foods from the clean list into your favorite meals, or give your old favorites a makeover. Here are some sample meals to get you going:

Breakfast:

- Smoothies: Create milk-based (i.e. almond, coconut, hemp, or even flax are the best) smoothies with organic fruits and greens. Feel free to add healthy fats such as 1tbs. of coconut oil or nut butter.
- Protein-Packed: Use pasture-raised eggs to make delicious and filling morning meals. I love a soft-cooked egg on gluten-free toast on occassion. Try a scramble with precooked vegetables, or maybe add a tbsp. or so of goat cheese.
- Oats: If you're eating oats, use gluten-free steel-cut oats. They cook slower, but they have a lower glycemic rating and are less processed.
- Unconventional: Feel free to think out of the breakfast box. I often eat a salad or even soup as my morning meal.
- Tea: Teas are great as they give you tons of antioxidants and really have no downside, and they are a much better option than coffee, which can cause over acidity.

Lunches:

- If you're packing a lunch, think lots of fresh vegetables, proteins, and something a little heavier such as quinoa or root vegetables like sweet potatoes, yams, beets, or carrots. These have more sugar, but as long as they are organic, you're eating clean! Whole, fresh foods are what you want. Precook as much as you can.
- Salad: Try a salad with quinoa, sweet potatoes, and goat cheese.
- Tacos: Chicken or raw walnut tacos on lettuce shells topped with lots of salsa are amazing!
- Soups: Soups such as homemade vegetables soups (made overnight in a crockpot) can be a quick and easy lunch
- Sandwiches: We all love bread, but it's not the cleanest or healthiest foods. IF you must have bread, try a gluten-free option. Then, start to wean off breads all together. Even if it's gluten free, it's a processed food.

Dinner:

- Protein: Any cooked fish, chicken, or beef in its whole form is acceptable. Choose wild-caught, organic and grass-fed proteins. Serve with your choice of vegetables. Get colorful with these!
- Soups: –Just like lunch, there are a lot of options: veggie, any protein, and not from a can!
- Omelets: These are great for using up vegetables. I love breakfast for dinner!
- Pasta: Pasta dishes should made from zucchini noodles, but the rest can stay the same. Try spaghetti with red sauce, pesto, or just homemade Italian dressing.
- Vegetables: Try vegetables as the main course, including baked spaghetti squash, sweet potato and bean tacos, serialized vegetable "pasta" made with zucchini, big mixed vegetable salads, roasted vegetables with goat cheese, and almonds.

Treats:

Try your hand at paleo baking. This pretty much follows the rules of eating clean. I love baking nut breads. You can use 1 basic recipe and add dried fruits, nuts, and spices to your liking. Here is my favorite:

Basic Gluten Free Almond Loaf

- 1 c. almond flour
- 1 c. cashew flour
- 2 tbsp. coconut flour
- ¼ c. ground golden flax seed
- ¼ tsp. sea salt
- 1/2 tsp. aluminum-free baking soda
- 5 large eggs
- 1 tbsp. coconut oil
- 1 tbsp. honey or maple syrup
- 1 tbsp. apple cider vinegar

Choose any of the following to add (optional): 1 tbsp. chai spice blend; 1/2 c. blue berries, blackberries, raspberries or other small berry; 1 tsp. lemon flavoring; 1/2 c. sweet potato puree plus 1 tbsp. pumpkin pie spice; 1 tsp. each fresh oregano, basil, thyme and garlic.

Instructions: Place almond flour, cashew flour, coconut flour, flax, salt and baking soda in a food processor. Pulse ingredients together. Then, pulse in eggs, oil, honey, and vinegar. Transfer batter to a greased loaf pan and bake at 350° for 30 minutes. Cool in the pan for 2 hours or longer.

Nut Milk

Drink this milk on its own or use it as a substitute for dairy in other recipes.

- 1 c. raw nuts or seeds (i.e. almonds, cashew, walnuts, sunflower seeds, hemp seeds)

- 4 c. water
- Sea salt
- Vanilla
- Monk fruit powder (optional sweetener)

Soak nuts or seeds overnight or at least 4 hours. (This is not necessary for hemp.) Drain and add to blender with water, salt, vanilla, and monk fruit, if you want it sweetened. Blend on high for 2 minutes, then strain the milk through a milk bag or a fine mesh strainer. This milk is good for 5–6 days in the refrigerator. It can also be frozen!

Suggested Shopping List:

- 2 packages of fresh berries (raspberries, blackberries, blueberries);
- Wild-caught salmon, white fish, and organic chicken breast (use hand-sized portions per person if you are eating meat);
- Cumin, cayenne pepper, sea salt, pepper, garlic, onion, fresh cilantro, nutritional yeast powder, and other seasonings;
- Broccoli, cauliflower, Brussels sprouts, mushrooms, onions, 4 green zucchini, 1 spaghetti squash, romaine lettuce (whole leaves for tacos), 2 bags or bunches of fresh spinach, kale, 1 package small Portobello mushrooms, salad greens, cucumbers, jicama, avocados, and dates;
- Lemons, limes, and 2 packages berries (frozen and fresh);
- Matcha green tea powder and bagged green tea;
- Unsweetened, non-dairy milk (almond, coconut, hemp);
- Stevia, Truvia, or monk fruit powder;
- Pasture-raised eggs and a carton of egg whites;
- Chia seeds;
- Raw cacao powder;
- 1 package of goat cheese crumbles;
- Coconut oil, olive oil, and sesame oil;
- Gluten-free bread;
- Powdered peanut butter, almond butter, hemp seeds, and avocados.

Detox the Excretory Organs:
Your Built-in Cleaning System

The body has several "excretory" organs that are designed to excrete a fluid or substance in order to clean the body. We will be focusing on the skin, kidneys, liver, large intestine and colon, and the lungs. Each organ can be helped along using things we ingest such as healing foods, herbal medicine, essential oils, and cleansing practices.

Why do we need to perform detoxification in our bodies? Even though our bodies are designed with these organs to cleanse itself (thus excretory organs are there), we are being exposed to a larger amount of toxins than our bodies were ever designed to deal with. Exposure to these toxins comes, in large part, from the foods we eat. Most of the foods consumed by people are highly processed are barely resemble any food in its natural state. They are also heavily laden with chemical preservatives, colors, scents, and other toxic ingredients. To top things off, we are putting these so-called "foods" into plastic packaging, which then sends toxins into the foods or beverages straight from the package. All of this has to go somewhere, and our bodies are just not designed to filter it all out.

In addition to the toxins making their way into our bodies via food, we have toxins in the water we drink. Even if you buy bottled water, that water is now contaminated with the chemicals from the plastic in which it is packaged. We also tend to drink beverages that contain sugar, caffeine, alcohol, or artificial ingredients such as flavors or sweeteners. The tap water that we drink or bathe in also contains many contaminants, including residues from medications, fertilizers, pesticides, and any other chemicals that make their way into our water supply. These chemicals are not intended for the body, and so the body has to filter it out somehow.

Then, there is our skin, which is our largest organ. We tend to think of this part of our body as being a barrier to all things. While it does protect us from some bacteria, helps to regulate our temperature, and performs other helpful functions, but it's more like a sponge than a barrier. We can absorb much of what we put on our skin. Consider for a moment all the things you put on your skin each day. This could be soaps, lotions, deodorants, perfumes, cologne, and other cosmetics. Most of these contain toxic ingredients, which then go directly into your bloodstream. We can absorb toxins from things that touch our skin, as well, such as clothing, plastics, flooring, and other things you encounter on a daily basis.

We absorb toxins through the lungs by breathing in air, including whatever is in the air. This doesn't need to be toxic air from a dirty city; the air inside your home is more toxic than any outdoor air due to the off-gassing of materials such as paint, carpet, and other fumes.

As you can see, we need to give the body as much help as possible to create a smaller toxic load and to help the body along with the detoxification process.

Skin Detoxification

The skin is the largest organ in the body and has 2 layers: (1) the epidermis, or outer layer, and (2) the dermis, the inner layer. The epidermis produces keratin, giving elasticity to the skin and melanin, which also gives it its color. There are also Langerhans' cells in the epidermis that produce antigens to support the immune system. The skin protects the internal organs, fortifies against infections, and stores water and fat. Also, it excretes waste and helps to build vitamin D. These 2 functions are important in the natural detoxification and immune health processes.

The skin is the first thing we see and shows us when there is a problem on the inside. For healthy skin we must focus on detoxification, proper cleansing, and supplementing nutrients to the skin cells. Using the following herbs, foods, and essential oils, we can help detox the skin.

Herbal Teas:

Consumed hot or cold, teas are a great way to use herbs to clean the body. Here are some of the best teas to drink for skin health:

- Red Clover: This is best as a blood cleanser, antibacterial, anti-inflammatory, antiseptic, and wound healing.
- Dandelion: Dandelion provides abundant vitamin A for healthy skin and is also high in antioxidants.
- Lemon Balm: Lemon calms the nervous system and is helpful for stress-induced skin problems.
- Rooibos: This is a tea from Africa often referred to as red tea or "redbush" and is one of the best teas to drink for skin health. It contains over 40 polyphenol compounds, which have antioxidant effects. It also contains alpha-hydroxic acid that promotes healthy skin.
- Green Tea: Also very high in antioxidants, this tea has a protective effect on the skin as well as a detoxifying effect on the entire body.
- Chamomile: This herb is an anti-inflammatory and antihistamine and can help calm irritated skin, even when consumed as a tea. It can also be used topically on a cotton ball for dermatitis, eczema, psoriasis, ulcers, and wounds.
- Nettle Leaf: This herb is excellent for providing silica to the body for healthy hair, skin, and nails.

Foods for Healthy Skin:

Foods that improve the skin are those high in sulfur (garlic, onions, cabbage), those high in antioxidants (chocolate, berries, teas, salmon), and those high in beneficial fatty acids (walnuts, sunflower seeds, coconut, avocado, egg yolks).

Essential Oils for Skin

Essential oils have the unique ability to penetrate through the skin, enter the blood stream, and even enter each cell! Putting essential oils on the skin benefits not only the top layers but goes on to help you on the cellular level.

- Geranium: It regenerates tissues and tones skin.
- Lavender: This oil supports healing and maintains healthy tissues.
- Sandalwood: Sandalwood promotes new skin cell growth.
- Tea tree: This is often used as an antibacterial and anti-fungal.
- Frankincense: Frankincense promotes cellular protections and is an anti-inflammatory.

Essential oils for internal use include lemon, oregano, peppermint, and frankincense. (Limit to 1-3 drops at a time for internal use.) These all promote skin health when used internally. You can apply oils directly to the skin or, for sensitive skin, dilute in a small amount of coconut oil or mist on the skin adding 2-3 drops of essential oil per 4 oz. of water.

Kidney Cleanse

The kidneys are a major part of the urinary system, comprised of the kidneys, ureter, bladder, and urethra. The functions of the system are more than detoxification; however, the kidneys play a major role in removing drugs from the body, releasing hormones, producing vitamin D, and controlling the production of red blood cells. Flushing the kidneys helps prevent kidney stones and toxic build up, which often happens as a result of inadequate water intake. In addition to water, adding in the additional elements below helps to strengthen the urinary system and supports natural kidney functions.

Kidney Herbs

Use these herbs as a tea or supplement to help clean the kidneys:

- Dandelion: This stimulates the flow of uric acid through the kidneys and increases urine production. Drink a lot of water when using dandelion.

- Corn silk: Corn silk has a soothing effect on the urinary tract and helps to tone the tissues, and it has been traditionally used for kidney stones and urinary infections.
- Goji Berry: These increase levels of antioxidant superoxide dismutase, help to nourish the kidneys, and remove toxins from them.
- Parsley: This vivacious herb helps reduce excess fluids in the body, flushes the kidneys, and supports kidney functions.
- Uva-ursi: This herb contains arbutin, which in the body converts to hydroquinine, helping to alkalize the urine preventing urinary tract infections. It also stimulates the activity of the kidneys.

Foods for Kidneys:

Foods that help the kidney include asparagus, cucumbers, black cherries, cranberries, cabbage, red bell peppers, garlic, and onions. These are all diuretic and/or anti-inflammatory foods with high antioxidants.

Essential Oils for Kidneys

To support the kidneys, use these essential oils applied topically to the upper portion of the lower back and bottoms of the feet.

- Lemon: Lemon helps dissolve stones and acts as a diuretic.
- Juniper Berry: These berries act as a diuretic, tone bladder tissues, and support the entire urinary system.
- Cypress: Regular use can resolve incontinence and excessive water retention.
- Eucalyptus: Eucalyptus fights infections and kidney stones.
- Lemongrass: This cleanses the urinary tract and prevents infections.

Liver Cleanse

The liver is the dumpster of the body; it has to clean and filter the entire body's blood.

Herbs for the Liver: (Use these as teas or in supplement form.)

- Dandelion Root: It stimulates bile flow and production.
- Milk Thistle: Milk thistle stimulates a generation of new liver cells and prevents toxins from penetrating interior liver cells.
- Chicory Root: Clearing the heat and toxins from the liver, chicory root promotes bile flow and is often used as a common coffee substitute.
- Turmeric: Turmeric is an excellent liver tonic and increases bile flow.

Foods for Liver:

Food for a healthy liver include: beets, dandelion greens, beet greens, garlic, green tea, avocado, apples and "raw" olives, and olive oil.

Essential Oils for Liver:

- Lemon: It improves all liver functions.
- Cilantro: This herb improves all liver functions, as well.
- Geranium: Geranium is known to stimulate bile production.
- Grapefruit: This fruit may reduce fatty liver tissue.
- Rosemary: Rosemary also reduces fatty liver and is used for bile duct congestion.
- Helichrysum: This stimulates liver functions, improves bile production and bile flow, and reduces liver scarring.

Lungs Cleanse

The lungs help to filter the air you breathe, expel toxins though breathing, and balance the blood Ph.

Herbs for Lungs:

- Lungwort, oregano, and plantain all support lung health as a tonic.
- Nettles: They are an anti-allergenic, decongestant, expectorant, and pectoral (helps improve lung health).
- Grindelia: Grindelia helps expel mucus from lungs and is helpful for asthma and bronchitis, colds, emphysema, and hay fever.
- Mullein: Often used as a demulcent (soothes irritated or inflamed lung tissue), mullein is an anti-inflammatory, antiviral, expectorant, and pectoral (helps improve lung health).
- Licorice: Surprisingly, it soothes irritated lung tissues, reduces coughs, expels mucus from lungs, and nourishes lungs.
- Thyme: Thyme acts as a bronchial dilator, reduces coughs, and expels mucus.
- Osha: It primarily works as a bronchial dilator, antihistamine, and expectorant.

Foods for the Lungs:

Healthy foods for the lungs include coffee, green tea, berries, apples, leafy greens, salmon, chia seeds, flax seed, and raw nuts or seeds.

Essential Oils for the Lungs:

The following oils should be applied topically to the chest and feet or diffused in the air.

- Eucalyptus: It opens airways, supports proper respiratory functions, and fights infections.
- Peppermint: As well, peppermint opens airways, but it can also expel mucus and act as an anti-inflammatory.
- Rosemary: Rosemary helps with various respiratory issues.

- Melaleuca: It is an anti-inflammatory, and it fights infections and works as an expectorant.
- Basil: Basil breaks up mucus congestion, reduces inflammation, expectorant, and stimulates immune function.

Colon/Intestinal Cleanse

The colon and large intestine are often trouble spots for people because of poor digestion. When food is not digested and eliminated well, there can be particles left in the colon that cause further health problems. Keep the colon clean with good digestion and regular bowel movements.

Herbs for Colon Health

- Kombucha tea: This tea provides probiotics and glucuronic acid for detoxifying the liver and intestines.
- Burdock: Burdock helps eliminate metabolic wastes through the liver, lymph, large intestines, kidneys, and skin.
- Cascara Sagrada: Often used as a laxative, cascara sagrada may be combined with ginger.
- Senna: Use senna with caution because it can cause cramping. You may also combine it with ginger root to lessen the side effect.

Foods for Colon Health

Aloe Vera juice, flax seed, chia seed, goji berries, broccoli, sweet potatoes, onions and garlic are all good choices.

Essential Oils For Colon/Digestive Health (Add 1-3 drops to your water.):

- Peppermint: Peppermint reduces gas and bloating and is an anti-nausea aid.
- Clove: This oil kills parasites.
- Cardamom: It can reduce gas and bloating and promote general intestinal health.

- Fennel: Fennel soothes the stomach, reduces gas, and improves digestion.
- Ginger: Often used for intestinal health, ginger is also an anti-nausea aid and can get rid of parasites.
- Marjoram: It is used for general intestinal health.

Beauty Routine Overhaul

We all know that the skin is the largest organ, but, remember, the skin functions much more like a sponge than a barrier. The pores of your skin are a direct link into your bloodstream, and anything you put on your skin goes into your body. Many people spend a lot of money on organic foods while putting toxic products on their skin! This is like having a beautiful salad and dousing it in greasy, oily salad dressing. It ruins the work you are doing to stay healthy!

You may think that cosmetics, lotions, perfumes, and toiletries are safe because they are sold at almost every market and drugstore in the world. Most people don't realize that the Food and Drug Administration (FDA) does not require cosmetic companies to do any real testing of their products before they hit the market. In comparison, European laws are stricter and, as a result, they have banned over 1,200 chemicals that are still used in the United States in most cosmetics.

Some sources say that a single fat cell in a healthy human being can contain over 500 dangerous chemicals that come from man-made products. These enter our body through eating, drinking, breathing, and, most often overlooked, our skin. The National Institute of Occasional Safety and Health found that 884 chemicals used in personal care products and cosmetics are known to be toxic.

Here are a few of the most toxic and most commonly used ingredients in toiletries and beauty products:

- Sodium laurel sulphate (irritates skin, corrodes hair follicles, and impairs ability to grow hair);

- Propylene glycol (implicated in dermatitis, kidney damage, and liver abnormalities and also causes eye irritation, skin irritation, and nausea and headaches);
- Ammonia derivatives such as DEA, TEA, and MEA (combine with other chemicals to create dangerous reactions and are known to have hormone-disrupting effects);
- Phalates (cause birth defects, reproductive impairments, and are often disguised by the term "fragrance");
- Parabens (a skin toxicant that causes cell mutation, disrupts immune system response, and prompts rashes);
- Fragrances (can indicate the presence of up to 4,000 separate ingredients, most of them synthetic and cause symptoms of headaches, dizziness, rashes, skin discoloration, coughing, vomiting, central nervous system disruption, depression, hyperactivity, irritability, and behavioral changes);
- Mineral oil (impedes the body's ability to detoxify itself though the pores);
- Triclosan (found in almost anything antibacterial and high risk and is similar in molecular structure and chemical formulation to some of the most toxic chemicals on earth such as dioxins, PCBs and, Agent Orange).

The best resource for learning about toxic skin care products and how to avoid them is the Environmental Working Group database: Skin Deep.

The skin can absorb nutrients readily. The best way to absorb is through oils, which also keep the skin supple. Carrier oils are less concentrated than essential oils and can be applied directly to the skin without needing to dilute them first. They typically do not have a strong scent and many do not have a scent at all. Carrier oils can be used to dilute essential oils for massage therapy and, in some cases, they can be ingested as well.

Most of the oils recommended are used in combination with other oils or to add essential oils to. Another use of carrier oils is as a natural treatment to treat or prevent wrinkles and other signs of aging. Carrier oils don't clog pores and are well tolerated by the skin, so they are frequently used in various beauty products or simply by themselves as a moisturizer.

Good Stuff on the Outside

The following information will help you decide what to include in your beauty care products.

Include aromatherapy in your daily skin care. Essential oils have medicinal properties for fighting infections, increasing cell production, and preserving your oils and homemade products. They often add a nice scent, as well. Essential oils have volatile qualities with protective compounds and anti-inflammatory effects. Here are a few nice oils for the skin:

- Geranium: This oil heals wounds, balances sebum (that keeps the skin supple), and is used for treating and preventing wrinkles, dry skin, bruises, and varicose ulcers.
- Chamomile: The oil of this plant helps clear infections, reduces inflammation, and increases the ability of the skin to regenerate.
- Frankincense: This oil helps reduce inflammation in the skin, clears any infections, and can be used to treat staph infections.
- Lavender: This popular oil helps to relieve pain, reduce inflammation, kill bacteria, protect cells from damage, prevent tumors, and helps to regenerate new tissue.
- Melaleuca: This is also known as tea tree oil and is excellent for skin "disorders" such as fungal infections, bacterial infections, acne, cold sores, cuts, eczema, infected wounds, scabies, shingles, staph infections, and warts.
- Bergamot: This oil is great for oily skin and inflammation.

Use plant-based carrier oils in your products such as almond oil, coconut oil, primrose oil, and others.

Clays and Salts

Clays are used to draw impurities from the skin, remove excess oil, and tighten the skin. Beware of over drying! They can also impart minerals on your skin that your body will absorb.

- Bentonite Clay: Bentonite clay has been traditionally used to assist in mineral deficiencies and to help bind toxins, making them more soluble.
- French Green Clay: It essentially "drinks" oils, toxic substances, and impurities from your skin. Its toning action stimulates the skin by bringing fresh blood to damaged skin cells, revitalizing the complexion, and tightening pores.
- Fullers Earth Clay: This clay is sedimentary clay that has been widely used as a skin-lightening agent and is best known for its ability to be applied as "facial bleach."
- Rhassoul Clay: Rhassoul is spa-quality clay from ancient deposits unearthed from the fertile Atlas Mountains of Morocco.

Salt in Skin Care

Cosmetic Salts are used to exfoliate the skin and add texture to hair, and they are also used as cleansers and toners, to eliminate odors, and even as mouth rinse and toothpaste. Here are some of the most common salts and their uses:

- Dead Sea Salt: Dead Sea salt is a nutrient-rich, extremely fine, and partially moist salt perfect for bath products and scrubbing blends.
- Epsom Salt: This may be used in bath salts to soothe, relax, and relieve sore muscles.
- Himalayan Pink Salt: One of the purest salts available for culinary, therapeutic, and cosmetic uses, Himalayan salt has beautifully formed crystals, which range in color from

off-white to a lustrous pink, indicating a quantifiable amount of 84 trace elements & iron.

- Sea Salt – This all-natural, solar-evaporated sea salt makes the perfect scrub, bath salt, or addition to your custom-formulated bath blends.

Herbs for Skin Health

Plants can impart their qualities on hair, skin, and nails when used both internally and externally. Start with these easy-to-use herbs and add on as you learn more about plants:

- Aloe Vera: Use this herb both internally and externally to heal and soothe skin. It generates new skin cells and can have a positive effect on the skin even when you ingest it. Try using a fresh aloe leaf when available or buy the plain aloe juice (for consumption) to use both internally and externally.
- Chamomile: Used as a tea internally and externally applied to the skin, it has a soothing effect and also helps with inflammation.
- Milk Thistle: This is considered by most to be the king of liver cleansers. Your skin reflects your body's internal health. If there is acne or rashes of any kind, then liver-cleansing herbs can help to clear things up.
- Nettle Leaf: High in iron, nettle gives you that healthy glow. It is anti-inflammatory, astringent, bactericidal, and very healing.
- Lavender: Lavender is an anti-inflammatory, anti-bacterial, and antifungal product and can be helpful for those suffering from acne. Its ability to balance oil production makes it a great choice for those with combination skin.

Tips for Healthy Skin Practices

Do dry brushing followed by a sesame oil massage. Using a large bristle brush (sold specifically for this use), scrub your body, feet to neck, in a large, circular motion. Do this with your skin dry *only*. You will notice your skin flaking off quite a bit. After about 10 minutes of vigorous brushing, use 2-4 tbsp. of sesame oil (or coconut) and practice the same circular motions while massaging the oil into your skin.

Get a body scrub or do one yourself using sea salts, oils, and essential oils as discussed in this section. You can choose any you like or try a body scrub from the recipe section below. Scrub your body, feet to neck, in circular motions using 1 small handful at a time to cover your body. Do this standing in the bath so you can rise off or soak afterwards. This increases circulation and helps to detoxify the body though the skins pores.

Try going deodorant free or use an all-natural deodorant like crystals. This sounds bizarre, but your body is supposed to sweat. Using antiperspirants blocks the ability to sweat (detox), but you can avoid body odors by taking liquid or capsules of chlorophyll.

Recipes

Super Easy Natural Body Lotion

- 1 c. almond oil
- 2 c. distilled or purified water, warmed
- 1 c. emulsifying wax
- 20 drops lavender essential oil
- 20 drops mint essential oil

Add wax and oil to a crock pot or cooking pot on the stove. Slowly warm on the lowest temperature and heat until the wax is completely melted. Add your essential oils of choice. Then, add Water and blend with a hand mixer until completely blended, about 1 minute. Bottle and label. Lotion should keep about 3-6 months unrefrigerated.

Dead Sea Salt Scrub and Soak

- 1-2 c. Dead Sea salt

- 2-3 oz. olive oil or almond oil
- 20 drops lavender essential oil of choice or combination

Mix all ingredients well and store in a wide mouth glass jar. Standing in the shower (without the water running), scrub your body with the mixture then lie down in the water and fill the tub to soak in the oils and salt.

Purifying Mud Mask

- ½ c. Moroccan (Rhassoul) clay
- ¼ c. water
- 5 drops essential oil of choice

Mix everything well with a spoon, apply to clean, exfoliated skin, let dry, wash, and remove all clay. Follow with coconut oil or other moisturizer.

Detox your Home

The air inside your home can be as much as 100 times more toxic than the air outside! This is due to a lack of circulation and also to all of the elements in our home that leave toxic residue and release toxic gasses into the air.

Formaldehyde is one of the most toxic gasses in the air in your home. It is a colorless, odorless gas coming from building materials such as flooring, cabinets, particleboard, paint, and carpeting.

Formaldehyde was first listed in the National Toxicology Program Report on Carcinogens (https://ntp.niehs.nih.gov/pubhealth/roc/index.html) [6] in 1981 as *reasonably anticipated to be a human carcinogen* based on sufficient evidence from studies in experimental animals. Since that time, additional cancer studies in humans have been

---

[6] National Institutes of Health, National Toxicology Program Report on Carcinogens (https://ntp.niehs.nih.gov/pubhealth/roc/index.html)

published, and the listing status was changed to "known to be a human carcinogen" in 2011.

Other of the things in your home that contribute to toxic indoor air include asbestos, treated wood, insulation, gas from a fireplace, smoke from any source, dust, and pet dander. Drains also may contain hazardous chemicals such as ammonia, sulfuric and phosphoric acids, lye, chlorine, formaldehyde, and phenol. As well, toxic chemicals used in the home affect adults, children, and pets. Household cleaners contain a range of toxic ingredients including artificial fragrances, phenols, diethylene glycol, formaldehyde, and petroleum.

Discard all plastic food and beverage containers and replace with glass or stainless steel. Discard all aluminum pots, pans, and cooking utensils and replace with stainless steel. According to the National Institutes of Health: "The primary source of exposure to BPA for most people is through the diet. While air, dust, and water are other possible sources of exposure, BPA in food and beverages accounts for the majority of daily human exposure. Bisphenol A can leach into food from the protective internal epoxy resin coatings of canned foods and from consumer products such as polycarbonate tableware, food storage containers, water bottles, and baby bottles. The degree to which BPA leaches from polycarbonate bottles into liquid may depend more on the temperature of the liquid or bottle, than the age of the container. BPA can also be found in breast milk." (https://www.niehs.nih.gov/health/topics/agents/sya-bpa/index.cfm)

Much of our clothing is manufactured with fire retardants, especially children's pajamas. Beware and replace any that you can. Remember, everything that comes into contact with your skin will eventually make it into the blood supply and remain in the fat cells. Try using borax as a laundry booster or non-toxic detergents and fabric softeners.

Clean your water supply. To learn more about your city water. Install filtration systems for your home drinking and bathing water. This can be as simple as purchasing a gallon-sized water filter for drinking. If you have the budget, then take a look at your entire home to see where you can install water purification systems.

Get your home tested for radon exposure. The U.S. Environmental Protection Agency estimates that radon causes about 21,000 lung cancer deaths in the United States each year.[7] While other estimates might be higher or lower, there is a general agreement that radon exposure is the second-leading cause of lung cancer after active smoking and the leading cause among non-smokers. Many radon-related lung cancer deaths can be prevented by testing for radon and taking the necessary steps to lower radon exposure in homes that have elevated radon levels. This process is known as radon mitigation.

Detox The Body Through Ancient Practices

In many cultures, detoxification is practiced as a regular part of healthcare and maintenance. Although, here in the United States, most people take better care of their cars than they do their bodies. Even though the body is designed to clean itself, we rarely give it the tools necessary to do so. The tools are the right, cleansing foods, enough water, and enough rest.

In addition, we put a huge toxic load on the body every day by exposing ourselves to toxins through our food, beverages, breath, and skin. There are many simple techniques we can employ to help the body detoxify itself. Below is a daily program that you can use repeatedly for improved detoxification of your body:

Massage:

Getting a deep tissue massage is also good for the lymphatic system. Treat your body well today and get a nice massage! This is a good time to practice hydrating the body because it can help with the lymphatic-clearing process.

---

[7]   United States Enironmental Protection Agency https://www.epa.gov/radon/health-risk-radon

Deep Breathing:

Today, practice deep breathing to clear the lungs through fluid released in the exhale. Deep breathing also helps to alkalize the body. Slow deep breaths help to activate the parasympathetic nervous system, which is when the body gets the chance to recuperate, regenerate, and heal. Deep breathing also increases oxygen to the heart and helps increase circulation, relieving congestion throughout the body. In yoga, cleansing breath is called Pranayama, and there are several ways to practice it. Start with the easiest, 3-part breath (Dirgha Pranayama). This breath encourages very deep breathing. Sitting up extremely straight or lying on the floor, slowly inhale air into the belly with your hands resting on the stomach. Exhale completely. Breathe in deeply again, this time expanding the torso out laterally. Exhale completely. Inhale deeply again, bringing air into the chest and upper back. Then, exhale completely. Now slowly inhale and allow the breath to fill the naval area, the trunk, the chest, and the upper back, completely filling the body. Repeat 10 times.

Oil Pulling and Tongue Scraping:

Next, we'll discuss 2 Ayurveda methods known as "oil pulling" and "tongue scraping. To do oil pulling, when you wake up first thing in the morning, take 1 tbsp. of coconut oil into your mouth and let it melt. Then, swish it around your mouth and in between your teeth. This can be done in 5 minutes the first time, working your way up to 15 minutes. This method is meant to pull toxins from the mouth into the coconut oil. Spit the coconut oil into the toilet or trash (not your sink because it could clog the drain) and rinse your mouth with warm water. Next, use a tongue scraper (found at most health food stores for less than $10) and scrape the tongue several times. Rinse and then floss and brush the teeth as normal. Tongue scraping cleans toxins that make their way to the mouth and settle on the tongue.

Sweating:

As mentioned previously, sweating is a great way to clean the body. Find and take advantage of sweating therapy as was done among Native Americans for its cleansing attributes. The best way is to spend 20 minutes in a sauna, either a dry sauna or infrared sauna. If you do not have access to any of these you can wear warm clothing and do mild activity to the extent it promotes sweating. A hot yoga class is a great way to detox via sweating as well. Be sure to drink salted water afterwards (1/2 tsp. Himalayan salt per 16 oz. water).

Enemas and Laxatives:

If constipation is a problem, then use 1 enema from your local drug store. This is a safe and effective way to move the bowels within minutes, but you should only do it on rare occasions. If you are having trouble more often, then you should really look at the foods you're eating and how much water you are drinking and using every day. Make sure you consume extra water after an enema. Over use of enemas, colonics and laxatives can disrupt your natural gut flora or good bacteria. This is precious material you can't afford to lose, so be very careful in your use of these.

Also, magnesium citrate, about 300-350 mg, can be taken at bedtime to induce bowel movements in the morning. Cabbage is also a great detoxifier, especially when fermented into sauerkraut as it contains glutamine. L-glutamine is an amino acid that is very beneficial for healing tissue in the body, and it can heal inflamed or ulcerated intestinal tissues as well.

I feel I must say a couple words about colonics. I know that this has been a popular protocol in the area of "cleansing;" however, there are a few reasons why I do *not* recommend colonics:

- Excessive colonics can disturb the natural flora that lies in the colon and is imperative for the health of your colon.

- Colonics can cause cramping, bloating, nausea, vomiting, and even bleeding in the colon.
- Colonics are a medical procedure that comes with possible complications such as infections and perforation of the colon, though issues these are uncommon.
- They can cause dehydration and severe loss of potassium in the body, which can disrupt digestive function, heart function, kidney function, and muscle contraction.
- Colonics can disrupt the delicate sodium and electrolyte balance in the colon causing sodium depletion.
- The colon absorbs nutrients but is unable to do so when it is irrigated with large amounts of water.
- There is little to no scientific evidence supporting colonics.
- People with inflammatory bowel disorders should *not* use colonics as they can seriously aggravate the condition.

Kidney Flushing:

The kidneys do a good job at cleaning themselves, so long as you drink enough fluids. Try this today: drink 1/2 gallon of the lemon and ginger drink (mentioned in a bit) and, in addition to that, consume kidney-cleansing foods like artichokes, asparagus, and watercress. D-mannose powder has been used successfully to treat urinary tract infections (UTIs) and can be included as a preventative measure for those that are prone to getting UTIs.

Rest, the Ultimate Healer:

Today is your day to rest. Focus on resting the body. This means you are off the hook today! You can rest your mind, rest your body, relax and even nap. Rest is the most powerful way of healing your body. During rest and especially sleep, your body can do all the cleansing and detoxifying work it is designed to do. You can also include many of the previous day's cleansing techniques on this day, as well. In fact, all of these methods can be done on a daily basis.

Recipes

Lemon Ginger Detox Water

- 1 whole lemon
- 1 bunch ginger root
- Fill a quart jar with 1 sliced lemon and 3 slices ginger root, then fill with purified water. Drink this water as much as you like, refilling the water but reusing the herbs. The herbs are good for 3 days, but keep cold.

Green Shake

- 1 c. fresh organic spinach
- 1 c. unsweetened almond milk
- 1 tbsp. cacao powder
- 1/2 tsp. sea salt
- ½ c. ice
- Stevia to taste

Blend all ingredients in a high-speed blender.

Green Detox juice

- 1 c. kale
- 1 c. cucumber
- 1 c. celery
- 1 c. spinach
- ½ c. dandelion
- 1 whole lemon
- 1 inch piece ginger

Run all ingredients through your juicer and drink.

Lemon Coconut Tea

- Juice of 1 lemon

- 1 tbsp. coconut oil
- Stevia to taste

Combine ingredients in large mug and fill with hot water. Drink on an empty stomach, morning or night, to help with liver cleansing and killing bacteria.

Roasted Beet and Goat Cheese Salad

- 1 bunch beets, any color
- Coconut oil to toss with beets
- 2 tbsp. olive oil
- Sea salt
- Goat cheese

Trim greens from beets; remove stems, wash, and set aside. Scrub and chop beets into bite-size chunks. Toss with olive oil and roast in oven at 375 degrees until soft, about 40 minutes. Let beets cool and chop beet greens. In a separate bowl, combine olive oil, lemon juice, and sea salt. Toss with beet greens and put on a plate. Top with roasted beets and goat cheese.

Chia Seed Pudding (colon cleanser)

- 1 tbsp. chia seed
- 1 c. unsweetened almond milk
- 1 tbsp. cacao powder (optional)
- Stevia or monk fruit powder to taste

Shake in a glass jar or blend in blender. Let it sit several hours to thicken. Adjust the amount of milk as necessary to get the consistency you want.

CHAPTER 5

Step 5: Using Herbal Medicine and Essential Oils for Wellness

Herbal Medicine

Herbs have been used for thousands of years as a way to provide us with health and healing. There are many benefits to knowing how to use herbs safely and effectively. People often visit doctors with viruses such as colds and the flu only to be told that they should go home and rest. While this is true, they can also use some of nature's gifts to bring themselves a bit of relief.

Although herbs can be very helpful as natural remedies, they are also a viable method for preventing illnesses. Herbs, along with a correct diet, regular exercise, and appropriate nutrient intake can help you reach a higher level of wellness!

How to Use Herbal Medicine Safely

Herbs have been used safely for thousands of years! Although it may seem that plant medicine is relatively new, it's actually quite dated, the first physical evidence dating back 60,000 years! Many of today's drugs have origins in plants like white willow (aspirin) and foxglove (digitalis); however, medicine has taken on a whole new meaning over the last 50 years. Still, we can use some of these simple plants for remedies to help us feel better, treat wounds, or prevent illnesses.

There are a variety of forms of herbal medicine. Three of the most common that you will find on the market are teas, capsules, and tinctures.

- Teas: This is the simplest form of herbal medicine. Teas are usually made using a tea bag filled with herbs, but they are also available as "loose leaf" or un-bagged teas. They are easily found in supermarkets and are essentially fool proof.
- Capsules: These contain just about any plant material with the capsule preventing you from tasting whatever it contains. This is great for some of the more bitter herbs. Keep in mind, you can't really tell what is in it by looking, so buy from reputable companies!
- Tinctures: These are liquid drops often based in alcohol or glycerin. They are fast acting because they bypass the digestive system, but they can be harder to take because some have pretty strong tastes. The glycerin-based tinctures are fairly palatable for children or adults.

When to use Caution:

- Pregnant or Nursing: If this applies to you, then skip on the herbs unless you have done significant research to verify that the herb is actually safe to use. Most remedies have alternatives if one is contraindicated, in which case, pick a safe substitute.
- Taking Medication: There can sometimes be contraindications of herbs and prescription combinations. Check with your doctor or with a drug/herb interaction guide before mixing!
- How to Buy Herbs: Buy them fresh or dried Online! Herbs are available fresh in many markets. You can also easily grow

herbs in your garden or in a pot! Good examples of these are rosemary, thyme, basil, chamomile, peppermint, and catnip. Buying bulk herbs online opens up many new doors for accessing herbs; however, you will have to know what to do with them once they arrive!

Recipes

Easy Fresh Mint Herbal Tea

- 1 c. loose packed fresh peppermint
- 1 quart glass jar with a lid
- 4 c. boiling water
- Stevia or raw honey to taste

Fill a glass jar with fresh mint then cover with boiling water and put the lid on immediately. Steep at least 15 minutes or until cool if you want it chilled. Pour over a strainer or hold the lid off to the side a bit and pour the fresh tea into another container or mug. Sweeten with your choice of Stevia or raw honey. This tea is excellent for digestive issues such as gas or nausea, motion sickness, fevers, headaches, and just to enjoy! This recipe can also be used with any other herb!

Easy Chamomile Tea with Bulk Herbs

- 2 tbsp. dried chamomile
- 2 c. boiling water
- 1 glass jar with a lid
- Stevia or raw honey to taste

Add dried herbs to your jar, cover with boiling water. Put the lid on to preserve volatile oils, which could otherwise be lost through evaporation. Steep 10 minutes and strain into a mug or other jar. Add your choice of natural sweetener such as raw honey or stevia. This recipe can also be used with any other dried herb!

You also can buy her herbs online as well, get organic if possible! My favorites are Star West Botanicals and Mountain Rose Herbs.

Herbs for Immune Health and Infections

Herbs can be used in a variety of formats to treat infections in the body and boost general immune health. They can help boost your white blood cells or fighters and help to prevent illness too!

- Elderberry: The juice and syrup of elderberry has been used for a couple thousand years in the treatment of colds, flu, and coughs. They help with asthma, chicken pox, colds, coughs, flu, fevers, sore throats, and most any respiratory infection.
- Echinacea: This herb is used as an anti-infection treatment and is best taken at the onset of symptoms or beforehand as a preventative measure. One of its constituents, properdin, helps ward off bacterial and viral cells as well as increases the number of immune cells in the bone marrow.
- Olive Leaf: This unsuspecting herb is the leaf of the common olive tree that produces olives and olive oil. The leaves contain oleoropein that dissolves the outer lining of pathogenic microbes, yet, it has no negative side effects for humans. Although it's not common to have any side effects, take it with food to prevent any stomach irritation just to be safe.
- Astragalus: One of the most widely prescribed herbs in Chinese medicine, it is used to bolster the immune system, helping the body become more resistant to invasive pathogens. It also inhibits viral replication, slowing down and preventing the spread of viral infections within the body. This makes its important to use it at the fist sign of illness! This herb is very safe; however, it is not recommended during high fevers.
- Garlic: One of the oldest remedies for colds and flu, raw garlic takes the cake and is always available. No wonder they call it the king of herbs! It can help fight infections caused by

staph, strep, and even salmonella. Garlic is a perfect remedy for congestion and coughs as well as sore throats.

- Myrrh: A natural gum resin known as one of the gifts to the three wives men. I is used as an antioxidant and for fighting infections. The easiest way to use this herb is in liquid drops, adding 30 drops to water or tea and letting it come into contact with the throat.

- Thyme: This simple garden plant packs a powerful punch! It has natural antibiotic properties as well as being an expectorant for helping remove lung congestion. This makes a great tea when combined with peppermint to treat even the most persistent coughs. The best part is that it is safe with zero side effects. Great for kids too!

Recipes

Fresh Garlic Toast

This is a great way to get some raw garlic in when you feel a cough or cold coming on. It is spicy and delicious!

- 1 clove garlic, crushed or minced
- 1 piece of gluten free bread
- 1 tbsp. grass-fed butter

Toast bread to your liking. Spread with butter and top with garlic.

Thyme Mint Tea for Coughs

- 1/4 c. fresh thyme leaf
- 1/4 c. fresh peppermint leaf
- 4 c. boiling water
- 1 glass jar with a lid

Fill the jar with your herbs and pour the boiling water over your herbs. Cover immediately with the lid to protect volatile oils! Steep for 20 minutes or more. Strain into another jar or mug and sweeten with your choice of natural sweetener. This is also excellent over ice! I gave this to my kids when they had whooping cough! It was amazing. Also, you can sub dried herbs if you can't find them fresh.

Herbs for the Digestive System

Herbs can be used for almost any digestive ailment such as gas, indigestion, constipation, diarrhea, and chronic disorders like ulcers. Usually, the essential oil content in the plants is responsible for the carminative (gas dispelling) effect. When you have bulk herbs or "loose leaf" form you can make your own teas using a French press. These herbs can also be taken in capsules or tincture (liquid drops).

- Ginger Root: Ginger is the panacea of herbs for stomach complaints. It is effective for nausea due to motion sickness, illness, pregnancy, and chemotherapy. It is also helpful for gas and bloating, and helps to kill parasites in the digestive tract. For best results, use the fresh root for digestive system effects.
- Licorice Root: Licorice root is a common remedy in traditional Chinese medicine, and it is a natural antacid. It helps to heal duodenal ulcers and soothe the intestines. Do not use licorice if you have high blood pressure, and do not use for more than 6 weeks without taking a break within that time.
- Fennel Seed: This seed is good for indigestion due to its gas-dispelling effect. It is especially good for gas that causes cramping. Use as a tea or take capsules.
- Cardamom: This herb is particularly good for helping with the digestion of dairy products. It has a nice flavor, making it a good tea for after dinner to help with digestion.
- Chamomile: This is a general tonic for the stomach and especially good for stomach disorders that are associated with anxiety or nervousness. It's great for morning sickness and safe to use during pregnancy. Also, it's excellent for gastritis,

ulcers, and heartburn. Use 1–3 c. of tea daily and be cautious if you are allergic to ragweed.

- Peppermint: This simple plant increases the production of bile (a digestive fluid) from the liver and helps process your food. It is also a great remedy for nausea and vomiting as well as helping kill any virus that may be contributing to the problem. Peppermint tea can be consumed as often as needed. The oil of peppermint plant can also be used for digestive troubles and ulcers when taken in a capsule form.

Recipes

Gripe Water

- 1 tbsp. Fennel Seed
- 1 tsp. Ginger dried Root
- 1 tsp. Peppermint
- Stevia

Add ingredients to a glass jar, cover with boiling water, and put the lid on. Steep 20 minutes or longer. Strain and add stevia. This is great for kids of all ages. Babies can use this for colic with sips from a spoon at room temperature.

Essential Oils for Health

How Essential Oils Work:

Essential oils are the concentrated, volatile oils from plants that have a strong scent, so they are often referred to as "aromatherapy." They are used to support and balance the natural systems of the body. In fact, essential oils support healthy functions of all organs, of digestion, immune system functions, skin health, healthy aging, and mental processes.

Essential oils are highly concentrated and can be used in tiny amounts to help support the body on many different levels. These oils support the natural functions of the body. Essential oils can easily penetrate the skin and some contain sesquesterpines that can cross the blood-brain barrier, enabling them to be readily used by the body and support healthy brain function.

Further, they are non-toxic when used at the correct dosage, and most oils have a very good scent! Essential oils are used in tiny amounts to support the immune system, assist the functions of brain, influence various systems of the body, and can be applied topically to soothe and support healthy skin.

3 Ways to Use Essential Oils

- Aromatically: Using essential oils aromatically usually refers to diffusing or otherwise infusing the air with essential oils that can be breathed in and detected by the olfactory bulb. This enables the limbic system and can assist brain functions that relate to memory and mood. Any oil that is smelled is considered to be used aromatically. It can be sprayed, diffused, steamed, or rubbed on the body or other items, such as fabric, where it can be detected by the brain. Oils diffused into the air can clean the air and help to eliminate odors. Diffused oils can also settle on the ground, where they might come into contact with feet as we walk on these surfaces.

- Topically: The skin absorbs all that you put on it. In this way, essential oils can go into the body and then penetrate pathogenic cells helping support the immune system. Every time oils are applied to the body, not only are the chemical constituents entering the blood stream and having their positive effects on the body, but also it is affecting us aromatically as we inhale the oils being applied. Remember that oils can be placed anywhere on the body can still go into the blood stream; however, the hands and feet have a higher capillary count, which means more "doors" to enter the blood stream. If you want to the oils to get into the bloodstream, go straight for the hands and bottoms of the feet. Applying essential oils to the feet is also a good way to use them with kids so that they do not touch it with their hands and mistakenly get it into their eyes.

- Internally: It is safe to use most oils internally in very small amounts. The oils deemed safe by the FDA for consumption are on a list called "Generally Recognized as Safe" (GRAS).[8] This use is best for digestive support, immune support, digestive support, and detoxification support. When using oils internally, limit it to 2-3 drops of an oil 2-3 times each day. Be sure to use only oils that are suggested for internal use.

Suggested Practice Activities

Purchase a oil that attracts you. Suggestions to get started are lavender, lemon, orange, peppermint, frankincense, or geranium. Also, look for ways to diffuse the oils such as an electric diffuser, candle diffuser, misting spray bottles, or even cotton balls to apply oils on.

Topical application. Patch test oils first. Try each oil, one drop at a time. Mix 1 drop of oil in fractionated coconut oil or grape seed oil. This is called a carrier oil. Using oils undiluted is called using them "neat." This will help to decipher whether or not you are sensitive to the oil.

Essential oils can also be mixed into unscented lotions and carrier oils to use all over the body. Remember to avoid mucous membranes such as eyes, nostrils, and genitals, as it can burn. If a oil irritates the skin, first use your carrier oil, like coconut oil, to remove the essential oil.

---

[8]   U.S. Food and Drug Administration. https://www.accessdata.fda.gov/scripts/cdrh/cfdocs/cfcfr/CFRSearch.cfm?fr=182.20

Do not use water to remove oils! This only spreads the oils, and if you get it in your eyes, it will burn. Use a carrier oil on a cotton ball then wash with soap and water.

For internal application, start with just 1 or 2 oils when using them internally so you can monitor their effects. Lemon oil is a great oil to use because it is mild with a wide range of benefits. A rule of thumb when using oils internally is to use oils that come from foods or herbs you might normally eat. Examples are lemon, grapefruit, peppermint, fennel, basil, etc. Always start with 1 drop to test it. You can always add more, but once it is in, it is difficult to dilute.

Recipes

Morning Kidney Flush

- 1 c. room temperature water
- 2 drops lemon essential oil

Natural Mouth Rinse

- 1 c. water
- 1/2 tsp baking soda
- 1 drop peppermint essential oil

Mix everything in a glass bottle with a tight cap. This is great for killing bacteria in the mouth, getting rid of onion and garlic breath and is much more gentle than mouthwashes with alcohol.

Sun Soother

- 1/4 c. aloe vera juice
- 5 drops lavender essential oil

Mix and store in refrigerator. Use 1 tsp. at a time on burns.

Scrape and Scratch Ointment

- 1/4 c. coconut oil, melted
- 5 drops melaleuca oil

Blend ingredients together and store in a refrigerator. Use topically on minor scrapes and cuts to disinfect.

Try any of the above recipes this week. Make notes on what you liked, did not like, any reactions to any of the oils, and etc. in this chart:

Oil Used	Form Used	Reactions	Notes
ex. lavender	diluted in oil	loved it	may blend with geranium

5 Basic Oils to Have on Hand at All Times

The following are just a few of some of the most commonly used essential oils. These are some of the most versatile and easy-to-use oils, but there are many more oils available on the market. Start by using a few of these then slowly add on to your arsenal as you learn and study the oils one by one!

Lavender is considered a universal oil that it used to work on almost anything!

- Supports Healthy Skin: Get too much sun? Lavender instantly reduces the discomfort from spending too much time in the sun and helps to prevent or reduce blistering, swelling, or peeling. This also works well anytime the skin is exposed to too much heat.

- Skin Irritation: Rashes, bug bite, abrasions, discomfort, and swelling are all taken care of by lavender, and it speeds the regeneration process. Apply 1-2 drops on the irritated area.
- Supports Natural Recovery Sprains or Muscle Soreness: Apply topically onto areas of discomfort.
- Supports Healthy Emotional States Stress/Mood/Sleeping Issues: It's commonly known to help reduce restlessness and help you sleep. It works by stimulating your limbic system. Apply to bottoms of feet or diffuse.
- Supports Headaches: Diffuse several drops or inhale mist or apply 1-2 drops on the back of the neck and temples.
- Supports Vascular Health: Have high blood pressure? Use 1-2 drops on back of the neck, chest, or taken internally in capsule form.

Melaleuca, also known as tea tree oil, it's used as a stand in (much better) for antibacterial creams.

- Supports Healthy Immune Functions: For candida and fungal-related infections, use internally in a capsule or apply 1-2 drops to affected area. For vaginal yeast infections, dilute 2-3 drops in coconut oil and apply to a tampon, then wear the tampon to bed and remove in the morning.
- *Supports Healthy Skin: Use it for cuts, wounds, and first aid. Use topically to clean wound. Dilute 1-2 drops or use undiluted. Acne, cold sores, and skin infections can also get relief. Use 1-3 drops topically to affected area.
- Misc. Uses: It repels mosquitos, mites, and ticks. Apply with a spray bottle mist with 1-3 drops per 1 oz. of water. It's great for sore throats infections of the mouth or throat, and gums. Use 1-3 drops diluted in water, gargle, and spit it out.

Lemon essential oil is made from the rind of the lemon and has many uses.

- Supports Healthy Mood: Lemon improves the mood and improves concentration. Diffuse 3-5 drops aromatically
- Supports Healthy Respiratory System: Respiratory congestion, allergies, sinus congestion, or runny nose may be soothed by applying 1-3 drops topically to chest and neck.
- Supports Healthy Digestion: Digestive health, acid reflux and heartburn may all be supported. Use 1-3 drops in water. Lemon oil helps the natural cleansing effects of the liver and kidneys, they body's built in detoxification organs.
- Supports Home Cleaning: Add a few drops to a cleaning solution, use 10 drops diluted in water, and spray onto furniture to clean and polish.

Peppermint reduces discomfort topically and internally. It also resists bacteria, protects cells from damage, aids in the body's natural inflammatory response, normalizes muscle spasms, and is very energizing! This oil makes a great natural mouth freshener as well and is great for gum and dental health. A drop of peppermint oil in water helps the digestive organs and reduces gas.

- Supports Healthy Stress Responses: For headaches, use 1 drop diluted in coconut oil to back of the neck or temples (avoid eyes!).
- Supports Dental Health: Peppermint can support dental health and freshen breath. Use 1 drop added to toothpaste or 1 drop diluted in water for mouthwash to freshen breath.
- Supports Respiratory Healthy Congestion: Diffuse or apply 1 drop diluted in oil to the bridge of your nose.
- Supports Natural Energy Levels: For energy enhancement, diffuse or apply 1 diluted drop under nose or back of neck.
- Supports Food Cravings: Apply under nose (diluted) before meals or inhale.

- Supports Fevers and Hot flashes: Apply 1 drop to back of neck or add 1 drop to water bottle and mist. Avoid eyes!

Frankincense is known for its ability to help with the body's natural inflammation response and to protect cells from damage. This oil supports healthy immune function, aids the respiratory system, and is very calming to the body and mind. It is often used for meditation and to promote rest. As well, this essential oil is excellent for promoting joint health, breast health, and women's reproductive health and contains many antioxidants that help fight free radicals making it an excellent choice for promoting healthy, youthful skin!

- Supports Mood: For mood enhancement, diffuse or take 1 drop under the tongue.
- Supports Healthy Skin Scarring/Skin Care/Wrinkles: Apply 1-3 drops undiluted to areas of concern.
- Supports Cellular Health: For cellular protection, take 1-3 drops internally daily or apply to the bottoms of the feet.
- Supports Relaxation Meditation/Relaxation: Apply 1 drop to back of neck or crown of head.

Using Oils in Foods and Drinks

Remember, essential oils can be ingested in small quantities as long as the oils come from plants that are on the GRAS list. Always use oils in small quantities, such as 1-3 drops, and dilute in foods or drinks before consuming them. This will help you to identify how the oil works for you and whether or not you should have any allergic reactions. Do not give children under 13 any oils to ingest.

Wild Orange Oil:

- Supports cellular health
- Supports healthy mood
- Supports healthy muscle and tissue recovery
- Supports digestive health

Wild orange oil is excellent for helping keep the natural digestive flora in check. Add this oil to foods and drinks in small quantities (1 drop at a time!).

Basil:

- Supports immune health
- Supports healthy respiratory response
- Supports natural kidney functions

Add a drop or two to pesto or other Italian sauces. It also makes a great beverage.

Cinnamon:

- Supports immune function
- Supports healthy inflammatory response
- Supports digestive health

This oil can be hot, so be careful if you use it on the skin and always dilute it! Try adding a drop to your tea or coffee.

Fennel:

- Supports immune response
- Supports healthy smooth tissue response
- Supports healthy digestive response
- Supports kidney and urinary health

Fennel is anti-parasitic, antispasmodic (relaxes muscles and reduces cramps), anti-toxic, and diuretic. Use this oil for stomach cramps, gas and bloating, gout, parasites, lactation, urinary stones, and to improve digestion.

Peppermint:

- Supports the body's natural healing capabilities

- Supports healthy digestion
- Supports healthy inflammatory response

Peppermint is analgesic, anti-inflammatory, antiseptic, and antispasmodic. Use this oil to stimulate brain function and increase energy, and it's perfect for improving respiratory functions and supporting the immune system, respiratory system, and digestive system. It's also helpful during times of menopause and PMS. This oil also makes the perfect and powerful breath freshener and kills bacteria in the mouth. If you are traveling and suffer from jet lag, peppermint oil can help to energize you! If you are congested or have a weakened sense of smell, peppermint can stimulate your sense of smell.

Grapefruit:

- Supports healthy metabolism
- Supports healthy digestion
- Supports mood

Grapefruit is an excellent aid to weight loss programs; it helps to quiet food craving and reduce bloating and water retention! As with all citrus oils, it's great for lifting the mood by helping you deal with stress! Use this oil for many types of addictions as it reduces cravings!

Use lime oil for improving your mood, helping you to cope with stress or melancholy. It supports the vascular system with blood pressure regulation, and it's great for adding to food as a natural immune stimulant and support for the immune system.

Oregano oil is extremely powerful oil, so be careful! Use it for stimulating the immune system, athlete's foot, candida, parasites, and warts.

Ginger oil is often used as a whole herb and is one of the most popular in Chinese medicine! It's an antiseptic, laxative, stimulant, tonic, and warming oil. Use it for diarrhea, gas, indigestion, low libido, morning sickness, nausea, vertigo, and vomiting.

Recipes

Detox Water

- 1 gallon distilled water
- 5 drops lemon essential oil
- 5 drops grapefruit oil
- 5 drops ginger essential oil

Combine and shake well before serving. Store in a glass container.

Lemon Hummus

- 1 c. garbanzo beans, rinsed
- 1/4 c. tahini
- 1 clove garlic, crushed
- 1 tsp sea salt
- 4 tbsp. olive oil
- 2 drops lemon oil

I use a food processor to make this recipe. Grind the garbanzo beans (you can also sub with peeled zucchini) until it is creamy, then add the remaining ingredients and blend well. Drizzle with olive oil and top with pitted kalamata olives if you like!

Peppermint Chocolates (Sugar Free)

- 1 c. coconut oil
- 4 tbsp. raw cacao powder
- 1/4 c. monk fruit powder
- 1 tsp sea salt
- 2 drops peppermint oil

Combine everything except oil in a pan, melt, and blend well. Add peppermint. Pour into cupcake papers in a muffin pan, 1 tbsp. per cup. Freeze. These will melt under 75 degrees, so keep them refrigerated.

Oil Used	Form Used	Reactions	Notes

Oils for Skin, Hair, and Overall Beauty

Essential oils have always been used on the skin and hair as a beauty treatment and for their scent. Oils used topically have many uses and are safe and easy for anyone. Try out each oil individually and always dilute them. This is a great way to see how the oil reacts with your body and your skin.

Geranium is an antiseptic, astringent, diuretic, insect repellent, relaxing and calming sedative. It is used in skin care is attributed to its anti-inflammatory effects that can help improve skin tone and texture. It is commonly used for calming nerves, broken capillaries bruises, dry hair (rub on the ends), low libido, hormone imbalance, dry skin, sensitive skin, varicose veins, and ulcers.

- Dry Hair/Dry Skin: Apply geranium topically to hair, scalp, and skin to maintain moisture balance.
- Deodorant: Apply topically under arms to decrease body odor.
- Cleansing: Apply topically over organs or take 1-2 drops internally to support liver, gall bladder, pancreas, and kidneys.
- Wounds: Apply 1-3 drops topically several times daily to keep wounds clean, promote healing, and prevent scarring.

Sandalwood is an antiseptic, anti-tumor, aphrodisiac, astringent, calming, and sedative oil. Use this oil for general skin care, moles, dry skin, dry hair, and for calming the mind.

- Wounds/Scars/Acne/Skin Care: Use 1-2 drops directly on areas of concern.
- Relaxation/Stress/Calming: Diffuse in the air or apply to back of the neck or under the nose.
- Alzheimer's Disease: Take internally to support immune function.

Myrrh is an anti-inflammatory, antiseptic and astringent. Use this oil for chapped or cracked skin, stretch makes, skin ulcers, and weeping wounds.

- Fine Lines: Apply 1-2 drops directly to areas of concern.
- Eczema and Wounds: Apply 1-2 drips undiluted to the skin or take 1-2 drops internally or in a capsule.
- Mood Enhancement: Apply 1-2 drops to the back of the neck.
- Gums and Teeth: Apply topically to gums or add to toothpaste to improve gum health.

Ylang ylang is an antiseptic, antispasmodic (reduces cramps and muscle spasms), and sedative. Use this oil as an aphrodisiac, for calming the nerves (and skin), and for hormone balancing.

- Hormone Balance: Apply 1-3 drop to bottoms of feet, take internally under the tongue or in capsule, or diffuse into the air.
- Hair Growth: Apply 1-3 drops to the scalp or combine with hair care products to stimulate hair growth.
- Skin Care: Use 1-2 drops directly on the skin to control oil.
- Mental Fatigue/Low Libido/Impotence: Diffuse and apply 1-3 drops to the back of the neck.

Chamomile is an anti-inflammatory, antiparasitic, antispasmodic, calming, and relaxing oil. Use this oil for bee stings, insomnia, menopause symptoms, dry skin, rashes, and anywhere skin needs attention.

Sugar Scrub

- 2-3 oz. olive oil or other natural oil
- 1-c. fine white sugar
- 1 tbsp. each lavender flowers, calendula flowers (petals only), and roses (petals only) (you can use any other herb you like as long as it's soft)
- 20 drops lavender essential oil
- 20 drops geranium essential oil

Mix all ingredients well and store in a wide mouth glass jar. Use about 2 tbsp. and scrub your body while dry, then rise in the bath or shower. Salt can be substituted; however, it may irritate freshly shaved skin!

Simple Anti-Wrinkle Facial Moisturizer

- 1/4 c. coconut oil
- 5 drops frankincense oil
- 5 drops geranium oil

Blend all ingredients together and store in a glass gar. Apply 1 tsp. at bedtime. Massage the oil into the skin in upward motions.

Supporting a Body in Distress

Essential oils have the ability to support the immune system while they does their job to resist illness, manage fungus, reduce inflammation, reduce discomfort, and more attributes that make them perfectly suited for supporting health. One of the things we can do to stay healthy is to reduce our toxic load. Many of the toxins we encounter are from the environment, and it builds up in the body. This is called bioaccumulation.

Any substance that accumulates in the body that is considered to be harmful to the body is a toxin.

Toxins come into the body via food, drink, skin, or air. Some sources include:

- Prescription drugs and OTC drugs
- Pesticides, herbicides, or fungicides
- Dioxins and PCBs (industrial pollutants)
- Formaldehyde
- Heavy metals
- Plastics (bisphenol A)
- Chlorine

Use essential oils instead of chemicals to reduce your toxic load!

Bergamot is an analgesic, antibacterial, anti-inflammatory, antiparasitic (kills parasites), antiseptic, antispasmodic, digestive, and sedative. Use this oil for calming the nerves, colic or gas, improving the mood, stress management, increase energy levels, and hormone balancing.

- Acne/Skin Conditions: Apply diluted to affected areas.
- Fungus/Candida: Apply topically or take 1 drop internally daily.
- Respiratory Infections/Coughs: Apply 1-3 drops topically to chest.
- Emotional Health/Mood: Diffuse and apply 1-3 drops topically to the back of the neck or the bottoms of feet.
- Helichrysum oil, also known as "everlasting oil," is an antiviral, antibacterial, antispasmodic, and expectorant. Use it for abscesses, broken blood vessels, colitis, dermatitis, detoxification, occasional pain, and tinnitus. As a detoxifier, it pulls chemicals, toxins, and heavy metals from the body.
- Wrinkles/Scars/Stretch Marks: Apply topically to areas of concern, blends well with frankincense.
- Varicose Veins: Apply topically to affected areas.

- Cough/Colds/Congestions: Apply topically to throat and chest.
- Heavy Metal Toxicity: Take 1-3 drops in water or capsule to assist liver function and heavy metal chelation.
- Bleeding: Apply topically as a styptic and to help blood coagulate.

Lavender eases discomfort (analgesic), which is great for all sorts of bug bites and stings. It is also excellent for soothing skin exposed to excessive sun or heat; use it immediately! Lavender is great on cuts and scrapes as well but has a bit of a sting!

Melaleuca also disinfects with no sting, making it a great choice for kids' cuts and scrapes. It can assist the body's immune response to most topical fungal infections. This oil has been traditionally used on bacterial infections, boils, canker sores, chicken pox, cold sores, cuts on the skin, nail fungus, rashes, warts, and just about any minor wound.

Eucalyptus is an analgesic, anti-inflammatory, antiviral, insecticidal and expectorant. Use it for asthma, bronchitis, congestion, fevers, coughs, ear inflammation, inflammation, jet lag, kidney stones, neuralgia, occasional pain, respiratory health, and sinus health. This oil is best diffused in the air or applied to chest and neck for respiratory conditions.

Clary sage is an antifungal, antiseptic, astringent, nerve tonic, sedative, calming. This is a perfect oil for hormone related issues. Use for abdominal cramps, emotional health, estrogen balance, hot flashes, insomnia, poor lactation, mood swings, postpartum, pre-menopause symptoms, and hair loss.

Essential Oils Detox!

We are living in a toxic world and come into contact with toxins on a daily basis. Our bodies are built to clean themselves though our excretory organs (internal cleaning system); however, a little help doesn't hurt! A buildup of these toxins can impair your organs and cause disease. Cleaning the body through natural cleansing processes, diet and essential oils can reduce the toxic load and support each of your organs. The essential oils stimulate each organ to do its job better and help to draw toxins, chemicals, and parasites from the body while protecting from cellular damage, viruses, and bacteria.

- Frankincense (cellular detox, cellular support, blood toxicity, brain tissue detox, heavy metals, nerve toxicity, and skin toxicity)
- Clove (blood, brain, liver toxicity, parasites, and intestinal toxicity)
- Geranium (blood toxicity, gallbladder toxicity, heavy metals, and skin toxicity)
- Grapefruit (blood toxicity, cellulite, gallbladder toxicity, liver toxicity, and xenoextrogen toxicity)
- Oregano (candida toxicity, parasites, intestinal toxicity, xenoestrogen and toxicity)
- Cilantro (heavy metals, kidneys/urinary toxicity, and pancreas toxicity)
- Lemon (cellulite, kidney/urinary toxicity, liver toxicity, lymphatic toxicity, skin toxicity, and xenoestrogen toxicity)
- Cypress (cellulite, liver toxicity, and lymphatic toxicity)

Pain Relieving Bath Soak

- 1 c. Epsom salts
- 5 drops lavender
- 5 drops Deep Blue

Combine all ingredients and store in a glass jar. Make larger batches to save time. Use 1/4 c. per bath.

Chest and Neck Rub

- 1 c. coconut oil

- 1 tbsp. beeswax or emulsifying wax
- 10 drops eucalyptus oil
- 10 drops lavender oil
- 5 drops peppermint oil

Heat oil and wax on stove. Remove from heat. Mix in essential oils and pour into glass container. Apply to chest and neck then wrap with a washcloth, t-shirt, or towel and pin in place to hold in heat. Use this for sore throats and coughs.

Oils for Your Home

If you are working hard to remove toxins from your food, your skin care and other areas of your life then it makes no sense to use them to clean your home. Many people thing they are making their house cleaner by using harsh chemicals to kill bacteria, yet they are only introducing toxic chemicals that are probably far worse than the bacteria they are out to eliminate in the first place. Go with essential oils and natural ingredients for non-toxic cleaning and your home will be a much safer place.

Recipes

All-Purpose Cleaner

- 2 c. white vinegar
- 2 c. hydrogen peroxide
- 15 drops thyme, lemon, orange, or lavender essential oil

Mix in a spray bottle.

Tile Scrub

- 1 c. baking soda
- 1/4 c. liquid soap
- 15 drops lavender or lemon essential oil (or both)

- peroxide (optional)

Apply to tile and sprinkle with peroxide. Scrub and let sit 30 minutes. Rinse well.

Disinfectant Spray

- 10 drops essential oil such as lavender, melaleuca, geranium, lemon, peppermint, rosemary, or eucalyptus

Mix with water in a spray bottle. This can be used on hands or anything you want to disinfect.

Window Cleaner

- 1 c. white vinegar
- 1 c. water
- 15 drops lemon and basil essential oil

Mix in a spray bottle.

Carpet Freshener

- 3 c. baking soda
- 20 drops essential oils of choice.

Sprinkle on carpets or upholstery and wait several hours or overnight. Vacuum off.

Floor Wash

- 1 gallon water
- 1/4 c. white vinegar
- 5 drops lemon or orange essential oil
- 2 drops liquid soap

Combine all ingredients in a bucket.

Furniture Polish

- 1/2 c. olive oil
- 10 drops lemon oil

Combine ingredients. Polish wood with a soft cloth and 1 tsp. of oil mixture.

Oven Cleaner

- 1tbsp. liquid soap
- 1 1/2 c. baking soda
- 5 drops lemon oil
- 1/4 c. white vinegar

Combine ingredients in a bowl to make a paste. Coat oven interior with the mixture using a paint brush or sponge. Let sit until dry then scrub.

Toilet Bowl Cleaner

- 1/2 c. baking soda
- 1/4 c. white vinegar
- 5 drops thyme, melaleuca, and lemon essential oil

Sprinkle baking soda into toilet bowl. Add essential oils. Scrub with a toilet brush. Pour in vinegar and scrub more. Let mixture sit in toilet for 30 minutes or longer.

Dishwasher Rinse Aide

- 1 gallon white vinegar
- 30 drops lemon oil

Pour essential oil into a bottle of vinegar. Add to dishwasher's rinse aide compartment.

Garden Pest Spray

- 1 gallon water
- 1/4 c. castille liquid soap
- 5 drops peppermint oil

Mix and pour into a spray bottle. Spray on soil and plants to repel insects.

Bug Repellant Spray for Home

- 8 oz. spray bottle
- 10 drops lemongrass oil
- 10 drops peppermint oil
- ½ tsp. liquid castille soap (optional)

Blend ingredients in the spray bottle, add water to fill up the remaining space in bottle, and spray around doors, windows, closets, or anywhere bugs appear. They hate these oils!

Tile Scrub

- 1 c. baking soda
- 1/4-c. liquid soap
- 15 drops lavender or lemon essential oil (or both)
- Peroxide (optional)

Apply to tile, sprinkle with peroxide. Scrub and let sit 30 minutes. Rinse well.

Essential Oils for Pets

Lemon/Lime/Orange oils are antiseptic and kill bacteria, so they make great natural cleaners. They also help to cut grease and can all be used as stain removers, to dissolve sticky residue, and to chase away insects.

Lemongrass is an analgesic, anti-inflammatory, antiseptic, insect repellent, and sedative. This oil helps to purify the air of pollution and bacteria. It is also a good surface cleaner.

Peppermint is antiseptic and antiviral, so it makes a perfect home cleaning disinfectant. And it's safe and non-toxic for all pets, too!

Soothing Pet Shampoo

- 1 c. castille liquid soap
- 5 drops lavender oil
- 5 drops lemongrass oil

Blend together and shampoo pets with this to get rid of odors, repel bugs, and soothe skin.

CHAPTER 6

Step 6: Holistic Skin Care without Chemicals

We know our skin is the largest organ of the body, yet we neglect to care for it as much as we do the rest of our body. This series will teach you everything you need to care for your skin with natural ingredients you can make at home while learning about what to avoid.

Identifying the Enemy (What You need to Know about Products!)

Everything we put on our body goes into the body via the blood stream. It was once believed that the skin was a barrier for everything, but now we know we can use the skin as a vehicle for absorbing medications as well as detoxification though elimination via the pores.

We can use this to our advantage by employing only pure ingredients on the skin that have beneficial effects. We can also help to clean the body by using drawing agents on the skin to remove toxic waste.

What to Avoid

Avoid toxic ingredients such as parabens, phthalates, preservatives, and artificial colors and fragrances, all of which can be very toxic to your health. Also avoid:

- Oils that are not made from plants such as mineral oil;
- Products that contain alcohol as these dry the skin and the goal is to stay hydrated;
- Sun exposure on the skin, which breaks down collagen and elastin and can cause sun spots;
- Food or drinks that break down collagen, like sugar, alcohol, or caffeine.

Holistic Skin Care Nutrition

Here are some eating tips for healthy skin:

- Avoid sugar, wheat, soy, dairy, and gluten.
- Do not eat from 7pm to AM (or an adjusted 11-12 hour period each night) as this is when your body detoxifies itself.
- Drink 10, 8 oz. glasses of water daily (and more if you drink coffee or alcohol).
- Eat the right kinds of fat: focus on omega-3 fatty acids and anti-inflammatories (chia seed, hemp seeds. flax seeds, walnuts, sardines).

You might wonder why sugar is so bad for your skin or whether or not it is just generally unhealthy. It is, of course, generally unhealthy, but it is bad for the skin particularly from an anti-aging standpoint. When you consume sugar, your body creates enzymes that break down collagen. Depletion of collagen is what causes wrinkling and sagging skin. So, skip the sugar!

- Make Your Own Products to Avoid Toxins
- Make small batches and refrigerate or share.

- Use plenty of essential oils to preserve products and make them more medicinally potent.
- Some basic recipes include natural oils, emulsifying wax or other binding agent, thickening oil, and aromatherapy.

Oils for Amazing Skin

The skin can absorb nutrients readily. The best way to absorb is through oils, which also keep the skin supple. Carrier oils are less concentrated than essential oils, and can be applied directly to the skin without needing to dilute them first. They typically do not have a strong scent, and many do not have a scent at all. Carrier oils can be used to dilute essential oils, for massage therapy, and in some cases, they can be ingested as well. Most of the oils recommended are used in combination with other oils or to add essential oils to. Another use of carrier oils is as a natural treatment to treat or prevent wrinkles and other signs of aging. Carrier oils don't clog pores and are well tolerated by the skin, so they are frequently used in various beauty products or simply by themselves as a moisturizer.

Good Stuff on the Outside

Use plant-based carrier oils in your products such as almond oil, coconut oil, primrose oil, and others.

We can benefit from the moisturizing effects of oils by applying them to our skin and also by taking them in as food. Oils are fats and offer energy, satiety, and help to lubricate joints, skin, and intestines and to absorb fat-soluble vitamins.

Carrier Oils

Almond oil is one of the most useful, practical, and commonly used oils. It is great for all skin types as an acting emollient and is best known for its ability to soften, soothe, and recondition the skin.

It is a truly marvelous carrier oil and is equally superb for addition to body-care products. Natural expeller pressed oil from raw almond kernels is exceptionally rich in fatty acids. It stores well under any condition but extreme heat will reduce shelf life.

Camelina seed oil is very similar to flax in appearance and properties, but it has a much more stable shelf life and is not prone to rancidity. This delicious oil can be used for food and cosmetic purposes and comes packed with omega-3 fatty acids, vitamin E, and anti-oxidants. It's great for the skin, hair, and eyes, and the nourishing properties are also popularly used as an oil additive for our animal companions' food. This oil makes an excellent choice for natural cosmetics and especially hair-care formulas.

Camellia seed oil comes from the *Camellia Sinensis* plant, better known as the tea plant. This plant and, of course, the seed oil has high concentrations of antioxidants and is known for its ability to protect and repair the skin. It also helps in the recovery of wounds and stops the proliferation of microbes, and it is also anti-fungal and helps reduce inflammation. This oil is considered a pain reliever and to reduce damage to the nervous system.

Argan oil is a rare and exquisite oil meticulously pressed from the fruit kernels of the Moroccan argan tree. Argan oil is rich in natural tocopherols (vitamin E) and phenols, carotenes, squalene, and fatty acids, making it a very luxurious oil. It absorbs quickly and is often used in skin, nail, and hair treatments to deliver deep hydration, strengthen brittle hair and nails, and prevent or reduce stretch marks. It's wonderful for use in lotion and cream formulations or may be used alone. It also keeps well when stored properly (in a cool place under 77 degrees and away from sunlight).

Avocado oil is an ultra-rich organic oil and a delightful treasure containing high amounts of vitamins A, B1, B2, D, and E. It also contains amino acids, sterols, pantothenic acid, lecithin, and other essential fatty acids. It is highly prized to those with skin problems such as eczema, psoriasis, and other skin ailments and other varieties make a lovely salad oil for dressings and condiments. Also, it's highly recommended to those with sensitive skin, problem skin, and other irritations that require vitamin rich oil. This particular variety of avocado oil has a relatively high viscosity and is marketed as high-oleic. Because of the relatively unstable nature of this oil, it is recommended that you use the material as soon as you receive it and store away from heat and light. Refrigeration is recommended but not required.

Shea butter is an unrefined butter derived from the vegetable fat of the karite tree. The first choice in natural skin care and fine body care products, our certified organic shea butter forms a breathable, water-resistant film and is the leading natural product for moisturizing. A wonderful base for cosmetic recipes or used as a standalone application, this comes highly recommended for those concerned about naturally healthy skin. Our shea butter is hand harvested, certified organic, expeller pressed, and is imported directly from the processor for cosmetic use only.

Coconut oil contains MCFAs (medium-chain fatty acids) that help to fight off infections. It's great for keeping skin supple, provides a slight SPF, great for cooking, and eating with as well. This oil is solid at less than 76 degrees. Try a 2-minute moisturizer! (1 tsp. coconut oil, 2 drops geranium or other essential oil, then mix in hands and apply)

Essential Oils for Topical use:

- Geranium: Analgesic, antibacterial, antidepressant, anti-diabetic, anti-inflammatory, antiseptic, astringent, deodorant, diuretic, emmenagogue, hepatic, insecticide, regenerative, rubefacient, sedative, styptic, tonic, vasoconstrictor, vermifuge, and vulnerary
- Frankincense: Analgesic, anti-fungal, anti-inflammatory, antioxidant, antiseptic, astringent, carminative, digestive, diuretic, expectorant, sedative, tonic, and vulnerary
- Lavender: Analgesic, antibacterial, anti-inflammatory, antimicrobial, antiseptic, antispasmodic, aromatic, carminative, cholagogue, deodorant, diuretic, emmenagogue,

insecticide, nervine, sedative, stimulant, stomachic, and vulnerary
- Maleluca (tea tree): Analgesic, antibacterial, antifungal, anti-inflammatory, antimicrobial, antiparasitic, antiseptic, antiviral, decongestant, deodorant, diaphoretic, expectorant, fungicidal, immune stimulant, insecticide, and vulnerary
- Ylang Ylang: Antibacterial, antidepressant, antifungal, anti-inflammatory, antiseptic, antispasmodic, aphrodisiac, cell proliferant, disinfectant, expectorant, nervine, sedative, and vulnerary
- Chamomile: Analgesic, antifungal, anti-inflammatory, antioxidant, antiseptic, astringent, carminative, digestive, diuretic, expectorant, sedative, tonic, and vulnerary
- Peppermint: Analgesic, antibacterial, anti-inflammatory, antifungal, antimicrobial, antiseptic, antispasmodic, astringent, carminative, cholagogue, cordial, digestive, emmenagogue, expectorant, febrifuge, insecticide, nervine, sedative, stimulant, stomachic, vasoconstrictor, and vermifuge

Starting on the Inside:

Diet plays an enormous role in how your skin looks; it's the "view" into your skin. If you are dehydrated, then your skin shows you. If you are toxic, your skin will show that too. The following is recommended to improve your skin:

- Eating high-alkaline diet improves skin.
- Water and herbal teas are better than dehydrating beverages.
- Eat foods that help detoxify the liver (greens, especially dandelion greens, beets, and beet roots, and herbs like milk thistle and licorice root)
- Include anti-inflammatory foods in your diet such as berries, nuts, and seeds.
- Include inflammatory herbs such as garlic, primrose oil, and chamomile.

- Include daily herbs whether through food, drink, skin, or supplementation.

Favorite Foods for Healthy Skin, Hair, and Nails:

- Cucumbers hydrate the body very well, reducing swelling and the water retention that causes puffiness in the skin.
- Rosemary stimulates hair follicles to encourage hair growth.
- Chamomile tea is an antibacterial, reducing stress that effects skin.
- Flax seed oil, evening primrose oil, borage seed oil (provides EFA) help to balance hormones. They also improve skin tone and texture. Beyond just essential fatty acids, they offer gammo-linoleic acids, and these help with balancing hormones.
- Garlic fights bacteria, and its natural sulfur content reduces inflammation that is visible on the skin.
- Hemp seed is high in amino acids that are used to build skin, hair, nails, and muscle tissue. They are also very high in minerals that lend themselves to beautiful hair, skin, and nails.
- Aloe vera softens skin and works internally and externally. Use it internally daily for a healthy digestive system. Use it on your skin daily to tighten and soften skin.
- Burdock root cleans the liver and removes toxic buildup from the blood.
- Lemon is a citric acid natural peel and removes spots from the skin, and it is a natural bleaching agent. Lemon detoxifies the body from the inside out.
- Oregano is an antibacterial, fights infections, and helps to clean skin.
- Chocolate, meaning real, raw cacao powder, has incredible health benefits due to its very high antioxidant content. This is more of a preventative food than anything, but it's also a nice treat! Add the powder to recipes, but be careful of sugar!

- Coconut, including the meat, oil, and water, lends itself to better skin mostly by supplying MCFAs. Those acids are anti-viral, antimicrobial, and anti-fungal. The oils are great on the skin as a natural moisturizer.
- Olives and olive oil, are great, but don't cook with olive oil! Heating this oil damages its healthful features. Use a small amount of oil on food after it's been cooked in salad dressing or even on the skin. Olives are great as long as they are raw and cured in salt water. Canned olives offer virtually no nutrients at all.
- Egg Yolks are also a source of biotin, a B-complex vitamin, which is needed for healthy skin and nails as well as vitamin A, which helps with tissue repair.
- Papaya include AHAs or alfa-hydroxy acid, which offer anti-aging properties. It also is full of enzymes called papain and can help to remove dead skin cells to help give you a glow. Eat the papaya and rub the skins on your face letting it dry 10 minutes before rinsing it off.
- Oatmeal contains mucilage that is activated with warm water. You will know this by its slimy quality. This is moisturizing to the skin and exfoliates, as well. Grind to a fine powder and add a bit of hot water to activate it. Spread on the skin and let it sit 10-15 minutes for a moisturizing mask.
- Seaweed is an ocean vegetable! It's loaded with nutrients and excellent for the skin when consumed as well as applied topically. Seaweed, when applied to the body, draws excess fluid and waste products from the skin. It also acts as a cleanser for dead skin cells and other impurities on the surface.

Recipes

Herbal Bath Bags

- 1 c. whole oats
- 1 c. herbs of choice (roses, lavender, mint, calendula, chamomile, etc.)

- 5 or 10 drops of essential oil of choice

Mix ingredients in bowl and fill a muslin bag tying tightly to close. Use in the bath to convert your regular bath to a giant cup of tea! Herbs provide skin benefits and oats soften skin.

Seaweed Facial

- Aloe vera gel
- Purified water
- Kelp powder (or other seaweed)
- French green clay powder

Mix ¼ c. of kelp powder ¼ c. French green clay powder, ½ c. aloe vera gel, and about ½ c. to ¾ c. purified water in a mixing bowl. Mix this until it's smooth then apply to the skin with a facial brush. Let it dry then rinse it off. This is a great anti-aging treatment that can be done weekly at home.

Deep Sea Herbal Mask

- ½ c. bentonite or French green clay
- ¼ c. kelp powder

Use water or flower hydrosol of choice. Mix powdered ingredients and store in a jar. To use, take 1 tbsp. in your and mix with enough water to create a thin paste. Smooth over the skin and leave on for 20 minutes. Rinse and pat dry. Follow with facial moisturizer.

CHAPTER

7

Recipes for Healing and Self-Care Wellness Remedies That Work

There are so many books on natural remedies out there, I don't think we necessarily need another; however, there are a few things that I have used over the years that almost always work, and I stick with them. If you make the changes to your diet, then you won't have much to deal with. I have been fortunate enough to keep my health on track so that I don't have most of these issues anymore, but if you are in the throes of autoimmune disease, they may come in handy for you.

- Fatigue: I know we fight naps, but they do help. Set your alarm for 20 minutes and give yourself a power nap. Yerba Mate has less caffeine than coffee but will give you a boost and is actually anti–inflammatory. Use peppermint essential oil and mist it on the back of your neck and on your feet or add 1 drop to a large glass of water.
- Joint pain: Use the Costa Rican cocktail (discussed in a bit): 1 oz. diluted in water, 2x per day. Try 1 drop of wintergreen on joints that are bothering you.

- Pain: Drink 30 drops of valerian tincture in water and rest. This is best used at bedtime. Valerian root is a mild sedative and pain reliever. It will usually make you sleepy.
- Constipation or Bloating: Use the lemon ginger drink then magnesium at bedtime (1200 mg).
- Headache: Use peppermint essential oil on the back of the neck using a cool damp cloth, and use valerian root tincture if you can go to sleep.
- Recurrent Yeast Infections (Candida): Use 1 drop of oregano oil on each foot at bedtime along with daily high dose probiotics (BioK, Natren, or VSL).
- Urinary Tract Infection: Use 1 tbsp. D-mannose powder 2-3 times daily plus oregano oil capsules and probiotics.
- Depression or Mood Swings: Use 5HTP as directed.
- Intestinal Damage: Take L-glutamine powder, 5000 mg daily on an empty stomach. This is very helpful for ulcerative colitis and diverticulitis.
- Skin Rash or Irritation: Use lavender essential oil, frankincense essential oil, and melaleuca essential oil, one drop of each diluted in water and applied to rashes or skin irritations.

Drinks

Yerba Mate Tea:

What tea kills bacteria, protects the skin, cleans the blood, improves weight loss, decreases appetite, balances intestinal flora, alleviates depression, and energizes the body and brain even though it has no caffeine? It's the South American Tea known as yerba maté!

I'm hooked on this tea for what it does! yerba maté is traditionally consumed using a metal straw called a *bombilla* out of a hollowed our gourd that it's consumed in; however, I make it in my French press and drink it iced! Try it and see what you think!

Costa Rican Cocktail

Being healthy never goes out of style! Learn how to make this Costa Rican cocktail that heals the body in so many ways. This recipe uses turmeric, which are a powerful anti-inflammatory, detoxifier and protector of your natural flora. This is a great drink for anyone suffering from inflammatory disease.

- ½ c. chopped fresh ginger root
- ½ c. chopped fresh turmeric root
- 4 c. of water
- juice of 1 lemon
- ¼ c. natural sweetener such as monk fruit powder or raw honey

Simmer roots in water for about 30 minutes until soft. Blend in a power blender and strain (optional), then add lemon juice and sweeten with monk fruit powder or raw honey to taste.

Hibiscus Tea Bottles

If you're having trouble getting water into your kids (or yourself), try making bottles of ready-to-drink herbal teas. This hibiscus tea is sweetened with stevia. My kids love to grab these cold from the fridge, and they're also way better than a plastic water bottle full of plastics residue. These cute bottles of hibiscus tea are yummy and medicinal. Use it just to drink, but reap the benefits of them being antibacterial, anti-inflammatory, claiming, good for colds and congestion, fevers, digestion and more. I make this with loose-leaf dried hibiscus flowers in my French press.

- ¼ c. flowers
- 4 c. hot water
- Stevia or monk fruit powder

Let it sit for a couple of hours then add 1/2 water or soda water a pinch of stevia or other natural sweetener, and hibiscus tea. It keeps all week!

By the way, hibiscus flowers are cheap, about $5 for ½ lb. organic online.

Stress Fighting Tea

Did you know that 77% of people experience the physical symptoms of stress? And what's more, 73% of people experience psychological symptoms of stress!

With so many of us hurting both mentally and physically from the effects of stress, it's time to learn how to battle it using our favorite weapon: essential oils!

- 1 bag chamomile tea
- 1 bag peppermint tea
- 2 drops wild orange essential oil

Fill mug with tea bags and hot water. Steep 5 minutes. Remove bags, add essential oil, and sweetener if you like.

Fresh Coconut Milk or Cream

- 1 white Thai coconut
- 2 c. water

Open the coconut and pour water into the blender. Scrape out all of the white "meat" and place in a bowl. Check to make sure no brown shell is with the white meat. Add to the blender and blend on high 2 minutes. This is your coconut cream. You can pour in ice cube trays and freeze to add to smoothies or use in any recipe that calls for cream. Add the 2 c. of water and re-blend for a more diluted coconut milk.

Hair and Skin Beauty Smoothie

Our hair and skin lose collagen as we age, but we can add some back in through diet and use fruits and vegetables that support healthy hair and skin. This is very filling and more like a meal!

- 1 c. almond milk
- 1 c. (packed) fresh spinach
- ½ c. frozen banana
- ½ ripe avocado
- ½ c. frozen raspberries
- 1 tbsp. Matcha green tea powder
- 1 tbsp. grass fed beef collagen powder
- 1 tbsp. hemp seeds
- Monk fruit powder to taste
- Blend everything in a high-powered blender. Enjoy!

Green Mineral Shake

- 1 c. fresh organic spinach
- 1 c. unsweetened almond milk
- 1 tbsp. cacao powder
- 1/2 tsp. sea salt
- ½ c. ice
- Stevia to taste

Blend the ingredients together in a high-speed blender.

Iced Mocha Latté

Although I drink mostly tea, I do like a coffee now and then, especially an iced coffee on a warm day. This one is less acidic using cold-pressed coffee, non-dairy additives, and no sugar.

- ¼ c. organic coffee beans, coarsely ground
- 4 c. cold water
- 1 c. almond or cashew milk (the recipe in this book works great)
- 1 tbsp. raw cacao powder (optional)
- 2 tbsp. monk fruit powder
- Dash of cinnamon

First make the coffee by mixing the coffee grounds and water in a French press. Let it sit several hours or overnight. Strain and set aside. You can skip this step to save time and just buy cold brewed coffee in the refrigerated section of any health food store. Mix 4 oz. coffee with 8 oz. of almond or cashew milk and remaining ingredients in a blender for 1 minute. Serve over ice.

Low Glycemic Meals and Side Dishes

Veggie Curry

My awesome friend Barbara delivered this homemade curry dish to me. What a nice treat! I'm so lucky! If you're not using turmeric yet, you need to start. It has been used for balancing the body's natural flora, which is especially important if you suffer from candida-related illnesses. Turmeric root is a natural pain reliever and anti-inflammatory, protecting cells from mutating (cancer) and helping with digestion so as to improve liver function. Eat some curry today! Curry is usually served over rice and made with potatoes, making it very starchy and high glycemic. Here is a delicious low-glycemic recipe that uses the healing and awesome turmeric.

- 1 c. white mushrooms halved.
- 2 c. green beans, trimmed and halved
- 2 tbsp. coconut oil or ghee
- 1 yellow onion, diced
- 3 cloves garlic, minced
- 2 tsp. ground cumin
- 1 ½ tsp. cayenne pepper
- 4 tsp. curry powder
- 4 tsp. garam masala
- 1 inch of fresh ginger root, grated
- 2 tsp. salt
- 1 14 oz. can dice tomatoes

- 1 can full fat coconut milk

Heat coconut oil or ghee in a large skillet on medium high heat. Add the chopped onions and cook until they begin to look translucent. Next, add the minced garlic and cook for 3-4 minutes or until it begins to brown. Then add remaining ingredients and simmer covered for about 10 minutes. Serve over coconut "rice" or miracle "rice."

Steamed Broccoli Breakfast Bowl

I remember the days of cold cereal or oatmeal and toast for breakfast. I figured it was normal to be tired all morning. How are you starting your day?

- 1-2 c. broccoli
- 1 or 2 pasture raised eggs (depending on how hungry you are)
- 1 tbsp. goat cheese
- Himalayan sea salt to taste
- Ghee or coconut oil for cooking

Place broccoli in skillet with ¼ c. water and cook covered until water is absorbed and broccoli is softened, about 5 minutes. Add 1 tsp. ghee or coconut oil, then add eggs and cook covered for 5-10 minutes or cooked on top to your liking. Slide everything onto a plate and top with salt and goat cheese.

Grain-Free Almond Bread

- 2 c. almond meal/flour
- 2 tbsp. coconut flour
- ¼ c. golden flaxseed, ground
- ¼ tsp. sea salt
- ½ tsp. baking soda
- 5 large eggs
- 1 tbsp. coconut oil

- 2 tbsp. monk fruit powder
- 1 tbsp. apple cider vinegar

Place almond flour, coconut flour, flax, salt, and baking soda in a food processor. Pulse ingredients together, then pulse in eggs, oil, honey, and vinegar. Transfer batter to a greased loaf pan and bake at 350° for 30 minutes. Cool in the pan for 2 hours

Strawberry/Raspberry Jam

- 1 bag frozen berries, thawed
- ½ c. chia seed
- ½ c. monk fruit powder

Mash the fruit or blend in blender or Cuisinart, add the chia and sweetener. Blend entirely. Store in the refrigerator for up to 5 days.

Kale Chips

- 1-2 bunches fresh kale
- 1 tbsp. olive or coconut oil
- sea salt or other seasonings to taste

Remove middle stems from the kale, then wash and dry completely. Drizzle with oil and massage, mixing well. Spread 1 layer on baking sheet and roast at 350 for 15 minutes. Sprinkle with salt and serve.

Vegetable Stir Fry

- 2 packages angel hair shirataki pasta or miracle rice
- 1 package Asian stir fry mix
- Optional protein of choice (chicken, shrimp, beef, or tofu)

Rinse and drain noodles, then set aside. Stir fry protein of choice with a bit of oil. Add in vegetables, cook for 10 minutes uncovered, and then cover the pot to cook vegetables until soft. Toss in noodles and sauce. Serve!

Flax Seed Crackers

- 2 c. golden flax seed, ground
- 5 c. water
- 1 tbsp. caraway seed
- 1 tbsp. sea salt

Mix everything well in a bowl and spread a thin layer on dehydrator trays or a lined baking sheet. Bake or dehydrate at lowest temp until crunchy. The oven takes 2-3 hours and the dehydrator about 18 hours.

Salad Jars Lunch on The Go!

Did you pack your lunch for today? We usually eat better when we plan ahead. Try stuffing your favorite vegetables, proteins, nuts, seeds, and dressing (dressing goes in first) into a quart-sized Mason jar. They're great for on the go and require no plastic!

Walnut Pesto Pasta

Who's craving pasta? I love pasta but don't really like the bloated, heavy, and tired feeling after eating it. This zucchini pasta is super light but delicious with basil pesto and walnuts, so it is incredibly good for you!

- 1 large zucchini squash
- 1/4-c. olive oil
- 1-c. basil
- 1 c. walnuts
- 1 clove crushed garlic
- 1 tbsp. lemon juice
- 1tsp sea salt

Peel and spiralize zucchini squash and set aside. Blend ingredients in food processor. Toss and heat on high for 5 minutes.

Sugar-Free, Low-Carb Muffins

Who's not craving hot blueberry muffins today? Can you believe this is still something you can have and stay lean and fit? Yep, it's true! It's wheat, gluten, and sugar free. Don't be afraid to eat clean.

- 2 ½ c. blanched almond flour (white)
- 1 tbsp. coconut flour
- ¼ c. monk fruit powder
- ½ tsp. baking soda
- ¼ tsp. Himalayan sea salt
- 1 tbsp. vanilla extract
- ¼ c. coconut oil
- ¼ c. water
- 2 whole pasture raised eggs
- 1 c. fresh or frozen blueberries
- Spray coconut oil

Preheat oven to 350. Line muffin pan with paper cups and spray with coconut oil. Using a Cuisinart or electric mixer, blend almond flour, coconut flour, monk fruit, salt, and baking soda. Next, pour in coconut oil, eggs, vanilla extract, and water. Blend well. Last, fold in blueberries. Spoon into muffin tins and bake for 25–30 minutes. Enjoy!

Coconut Lime Cauliflower Rice

This actually keeps pretty well and works well for a packed lunch

- 1 head cauliflower, grated
- ½ can full fat coconut milk (or make fresh)
- 1 tsp. sea salt
- ½ tsp. hot chili oil

- 1 tsp. fresh grated ginger root
- Coconut oil for cooking
- Lime essential oil
- Fresh cilantro

Grate 1 head cauliflower into a pan with 2 tbsp. coconut oil. Cook on high for 5 minutes. Add 1/2 c. fresh or canned full-fat coconut milk, 1 tsp. tea salt, 1/2 tsp. hot chili oil, 1 tsp. grated ginger, and 1 drop lime essential oil. Sprinkle with cilantro and serve hot!

Spaghetti Squash and Eggs

I'm really not a fan of the rain, especially where I live, which is by the beach. It gets cold! The good thing about rain, though, is cooking! It always makes me want to cook something warm and delicious. Since I love spaghetti squash, I'm always cooking it and always have some ready in the fridge.

- 1 whole spaghetti squash
- 2 large pasture raised eggs
- Himalayan sea sat
- Ghee or coconut oil for cooking

Just add a little ghee or coconut oil to a hot pan and make a nest with your squash, then add a pasture-raised egg to the center and pink sea salt. Cook covered on medium high until the white is cooked and yolk soft.

Grapefruit Avocado Salad

I love this combo for a brunch salad, or anytime, really. Lemon, lime, and grapefruit are low in sugar and are perfect for following a low glycemic diet to keep blood sugar balanced.

- 1 c. watercress or spinach
- ½ c. peeled orange segments

- ½ c. peeled grapefruit segments
- ½ avocado sliced
- 1 tbsp. lemon juice
- 1 tbsp. olive or grape seed oil
- Himalayan sea salt to taste

Toss greens with lemon juice, oil, and salt and plate. Top with oranges, grapefruits, and avocados. Yum!

Roasted Beet and Goat Cheese Salad

- 1 bunch beets, any color
- Coconut oil to toss with beets
- 2 tbsp. olive oil
- Sea salt
- Goat cheese

Trim greens from beets; remove stems, wash, and set aside. Scrub and chop beets into bite-sized chunks. Then, toss with olive oil and roast in the oven at 375 degrees until soft, which will take about 40 minutes. Let beets cool. Chop beet greens. In a separate bowl, combine olive oil, lemon juice, and sea salt. Toss with beet greens and put on a plate. Top with roasted beets and goat cheese.

Collard Veggie Wrap

- 1 bunch collard green leaves, washed, and de-stemmed
- Sliced vegetables of your choice:
- Avocados
- Zucchini hummus
- Guacamole

Spread collard leaf with hummus or guacamole then layer with sliced vegetables and top with avocado. Roll and eat like a burrito.

Mexican Cabbage Soup

- 1/2 head of cabbage
- 1 chopped onion
- 1 clove garlic
- 2 stalks celery chopped
- 2 large carrots sliced
- 3 tomatoes diced
- 6 c. veggie broth
- 1 avocado
- Fresh cilantro
- Optional: chopped organic chicken or organic ground turkey meat

Cook onion and meat, if using protein with oil until vegetables are soft. Add broth and simmer covered for 30 minutes. When vegetables are soft, scoop 1 c. into a dish and top with salsa and 1/2 an avocado and fresh cilantro.

Zucchini Garlic Hummus

- 2 c. peeled and chopped zucchini
- ¼ c. olive oil
- 1 tsp. sea salt
- ½ c. tahini paste
- 2 cloves crushed garlic
- 1/4 tsp. paprika
- 1/4 tsp. cumin

Blend all ingredients in the blender or food processor on high until creamy. Then, chill in the refrigerator for at least 1 hour. Use as a dip or spread for wraps and sushi

Daikon Miso Soup

- 1 6-inch daikon radish sprialized or julienne

- 1/2 c. sliced mushrooms
- 1/2 c. purple cabbage
- ¼ c. fresh cilantro
- 2 tbsp. miso paste
- 3 c. boiling water
- ¼ c. lime juice
- 1 minced garlic
- Dash of hot chili oil

Prep vegetables and mix in a large bowl, then set aside. In a pan, whisk water, miso, lime juice, garlic, and chili oil until hot. Toss with vegetables and serve.

Creamy Cauliflower Soup

- 1 chopped onion
- Coconut oil or ghee
- 1 head coarsely chopped cauliflower
- 4 c. veggie broth

Cook onions with oil, then add cauliflower. Cover and simmer until everything is soft, about 20 minutes. Puree with a hand mixer or in blender, and then serve with a dash of coarse sea salt.

Raw Breakfast Pudding

- 1 chopped apple
- 1/2 sliced banana
- ½ c. blueberries
- ¼ c. walnuts or slivered almonds

Layer all ingredients in a bowl and serve with almond milk

Raw Tacos

You can use romaine lettuce or green cabbage leaves stuffed with either organic chicken or walnut pate to make a super yummy and 1 c. walnuts

- 1 tsp. soy sauce
- 1 tsp. garlic powder
- 1/2 tsp. cumin
- 1/2 tsp. chipotle seasoning

Grind the walnuts in a food processor until you have a grainy texture similar to hamburger. Mix in the remaining ingredients blending well. Fill cabbage or lettuce leaves with walnut mixture. Top with avocado slices, tomatoes, sprouts, and salsa.

Steamed Veggie Quinoa Bowl

- 1/2 c. cooked quinoa,
- 1/2 c. steamed broccoli
- 1/2 c. steamed red pepper
- 1/2 c. steamed sliced carrots (or same vegetables from stir fry) 1/2 avocado and Braggs Amino acids to taste!

Layer vegetables on top of quinoa, then top with avocado and brags. Yum!

Home-Made Sauerkraut

This is probably one of the most healing foods you can ingest. I just can't say enough good things about homemade sauerkraut. The cabbage contains an amino acid, L-Glutamine, which helps to repair tissues. This is especially important for people with gut issues like leaky guy, Crohn's disease, or ulcerative colitis. It also contains a great deal of live bacteria, the ones you need to reestablish healthy balance in your gut! Eat this often!

- 5 lbs. cabbage (green or red)
- 2-3 tbsp. sea salt (optional)
- Optional: caraway seeds, fennel seeds, dill, shredded carrots, dulse, chili peppers, cumin seeds, and turmeric

Thinly slice the cabbage and place into a large mixing bowl. Sprinkle in the salt and begin to massage the cabbage. Continue massaging so that the salt begins to pull the liquid from the cabbage. This liquid will become your brine, which acts as a barrier against any unsavory bacteria during the fermentation process. Work in any of your optional ingredients and the optional starter. When the cabbage is nicely wilted and a lot of liquid begins pooling around it, begin packing it into a large glass jar or fermentation crock. Be sure to push the cabbage down forcefully with your fist or a tamper/mallet/etc. This will continue to create more brine. Once all the cabbage is in the fermenting vessel, pour the brine in and place a clean rock or heavy jar on top of the cabbage (we used a small bottle filled with water), then cover the jar with a cloth or towel. Label it somehow with the date you started it, then store in a dark area of your home. Allow the mixture to ferment for 10 days to 3 weeks, depending on your preferences. The longer it goes, the softer the cabbage will get and the more good bacteria will be present.

Mexican Quinoa Bowl

- 1/2 c quinoa
- ¼ c. chopped cucumber
- ¼ copped tomato
- ¼ c. chopped red onion
- ¼ c. chopped or sliced avocado
- 1 tbsp. minced jalapenos or banana peppers
- 1 tsp. chopped cilantro
- 1 tbsp. lime juice
- ¼ c pepitas
- ¼ c. salsa

Layer ingredients in a bowl and eat immediately!

Dips, Dressings, and Snacks

Dairy-Free Milks, Cheese, and Ice Cream

Dairy products have been pushed as a source of protein, calcium, and vitamin D for more than 50 years; however, research has proven that we not only get more diseases from drinking milk and consuming dairy (obesity, heart disease and inflammatory conditions), but we also miss out on the exact nutrients they are intended to provide. Dairy products have the nutrients added to them; they are not naturally occurring. As such, it is more difficult for the body to absorb those nutrients, especially when there is an inflammatory bowel disorder (common with dairy consumption)

The use of nuts as replacement dairy products is a good way to obtain the nutrients we are looking for in diary (calcium, magnesium, and pmega-3 fatty acids) with no cholesterol and no toxic residue if you are using organic ingredients. Still, nuts are high in fat, so use these products sparingly as you would any high-fat, high-calorie food.

All nut-based recipes include a soaking time before using them. This is to eliminate the phytic acid present in all nuts and seeds, which can inhibit the absorption of minerals iron, zinc, and calcium in the foods you consume with it.

Simple Nut Cheese Wheel

- 1 c. cashews, pine nuts, or almonds (soaked, drained, and skins removed)
- 3/4 c. water
- 2 tbsp. olive oil
- 3 tbsp. lemon juice
- 1 clove garlic
- Pinch Himalayan salt
- Optional 1 tsp. probiotic powder

Soak almonds overnight in water. Drain and pop off skins. Place all ingredients in food processor and process until smooth. This will take a bit of time, so don't rush. Place nut mixture in nut-milk bag or colander lined with cheesecloth. Give a light squeeze and place in the refrigerator overnight to set up. You can use the cheese at this point or, if you want it firmer, place it in the dehydrator for 6+ hours (at 115 degrees) to form a rind.

Cashew Cream Cheese

- 2 c. cashews, soaked 4 hours
- 1 tsp. probiotic powder
- Approximately ½ c. water
- 2 tsp. nutritional yeast
- ½ tsp. sea salt

Drain and rinse the cashews. In a blender, combine the cashews and probiotic powder. Blend the cashews adding water as necessary, just enough to get is super smooth. In a strainer lined with cheesecloth, allow the cashew cheese to ferment for 24 hours. Pick a warm place, like inside your oven with the light on or the top of your refrigerator, to promote the fermentation further. Stir in the nutritional yeast and sea salt.

Oil Free Avocado Dressing

I love this creamy dressing for my salads and zucchini noodles. You can also use it as a dip with vegetables.

- 1 whole cucumber peeled and chopped
- 1 small zucchini squash peeled and chopped
- ½ large avocado, peeled and pitted
- Juice of 2 lemons
- 1 clove garlic
- ½ tsp. Celtic or Himalayan sea salt
- ½ tsp. chipotle seasoning (or other spice of our choice)

Blend all ingredients in the blender until creamy. Use within 4 days.

Raspberry Chia Jam

This is jam with no sugar, tons of fiber and anti-inflammatory omega-3 fatty acids.

- 1 bag frozen raspberries, thawed
- ¼ c. chia seeds
- 2 tbsp.–¼ c. monk fruit powder (optional)

Mix all ingredients well in a bowl and chill in the refrigerator for 30 minutes or longer. Mixture will thicken for several hours. Use on toast, desserts, or eat with a spoon!

Home-Made Protein Power Bars

- 1 c. almond butter or peanut butter
- 1/2 c. plant based protein powder (optional)
- 1/2 c hemp seeds
- 1/4 c slivered almonds
- 1/4-c. cacao nibs or chocolate chips (optional)
- 2 tbsp. maple syrup
- 1 tsp. Himalayan sea salt

Blend 1 c. almond butter, protein powder, maple syrup, and sea salt into a thick dough. Add remaining ingredients and blend well, then press into a square and slice. Store in the refrigerator or freezer!

Beauty and Self Care

Your skin is your largest organ and needs to get fed just like the rest of the body. While most of that comes from what we ingest, a lot also comes from what we absorb. Everything you put on your skin can make its way to your bloodstream, so if you wouldn't eat it, I would question putting in on your skin. Stick with safe and natural ingredients!

Fast and Easy Anti-Wrinkle Cream

Essential oils protect the skin and cells from damage, as well as reduce inflammation and in this way help to stave off wrinkles. I like to use this every night before bed and, sometimes, as my first thing in the morning to freshen up my face before exercising.

- 2 oz. melted coconut oil
- 10 drops geranium essential oil
- 10 drops frankincense essential oil

Melt oil slowly, add essential oils, and mix well. Use a small amount on your face, patting it under and around eyes gently.

Deserts

Pumpkin Pie

Shell:
- 2 c. almond flour
- 1 egg white
- 1 tbsp. monk fruit
- 1 tsp sea salt

Filling:
- 1 can pumpkin puree
- 1 c. coconut creamer (sub half and half or homemade almond cream)
- ¾ c. monk fruit powder
- 2 eggs
- 1 tbsp. pumpkin pie spice
- ¼ tsp. clove (extra)
- ¼ tsp. sea salt

Grind shell ingredients in the food processor until it forms a dough. Press into pie pan. Bake 375 for 30 minutes or until browned.

Remove and cool. Then, blend filling ingredients in the food processor and pour into cooled shell. Bake at 357 degrees for 50 minutes.

Pecan Truffles

- 2 c. raw pecan pieces
- ½ tsp. sea salt
- 1 tbsp. nutmeg
- ½ c. monk fruit powder

Grind pecans and salt to make a soft dough. Roll into pieces that are 1 tbsp. each. Dust with cacao powder or roll in coconut shreds. This recipe can be made in several variations, just substitute the spice and/or coating. Try cacao, carob, cacao nib, cinnamon, essential oils, ginger, etc. You can also add dried fruits; however, they will add sugar content. For cream-filled truffles, just puree half the above ingredients with ¼ c. water. Roll into balls and press a hole into the top of each. Add a dollop of the cream to each of the balls. Chill and serve.

Chocolate Peanut Butter Cups

- 1 bag Lilly's Sugar-Free Chocolate Chips
- 1 c. prepared powdered peanut butter
- Paper muffin cups

Prepare peanut butter according to the instructions. Set aside. Slowly melt chocolate chips on the lowest temperature. Pour 1 tsp. chocolate into the bottom of the tin. Shake to disperse and flatten. Chill in freezer 5 minutes. Add 1 tsp. of peanut butter to cooled chocolate. Then, top with 1-2 tsp. more melted chocolate. Shake to disperse. Refreeze. Keep refrigerated.

Home-Made Chocolates

- ½ c. coconut oil or cocoa butter, melted
- ½ c. raw cacao powder

- ½ c. monk fruit powder
- 1 tsp. sea salt
- Optional: nuts, cacao nibs, shredded coconut, dried berries, or spices

Melt all ingredients together on low heat. Pour into muffin cups or molds. Keep frozen!

Coconut Ice Cream

- 1 batch coconut cream (or 1 can full fat coconut milk)
- 2 tbsp. lecithin granules
- 1 tsp. vanilla extract
- ¼ tsp. sea salt
- Unsweetened shredded coconut (optional)

Blend all ingredients in the blender, pour into an ice cream maker, and follow instructions on the ice cream maker.

Sugar-Free Vanilla Ice Cream

- 4 c. almond milk made with ½ the water (thicker milk)
- 2 tbsp. lecithin granules
- 1 tsp. vanilla
- ¼ tsp. sea salt
- ½ c. monk fruit powder

Blend ingredients in the blender and freeze in an ice cream maker. Optional ingredients: berries, cacao nibs, finely chopped nuts, shredded coconut, and cacao powder.

Home-Made Chocolate Ice Cream

- 4 c. nut milk made with ½ the water (thicker milk)
- 2 tbsp. lecithin granules
- 2 tbsp. raw cacao powder
- 1 tsp. vanilla

- ¼ tsp. sea salt
- ½ c. monk fruit powder

Blend ingredients in the blender, then follow the ice cream maker instructions. Optional ingredients: various natural flavorings, berries, cacao nibs, finely chopped nuts, shredded coconut, and cacao powder.

Chia Seed Pudding

- 1 tbsp. chia seed
- 1 c. unsweetened almond milk
- 1 tbsp. cacao powder (optional)
- Stevia or monk fruit powder to taste

Shake in a glass jar or blend in a blender. Let it sit several hours to thicken. Adjust the amount of milk as necessary to get the consistency you want.

Avocado Pudding

- 1 whole ripe avocado pureed
- 2-3 dates (or 2 tbsp. monk fruit powder)
- 1/4 tsp. sea salt
- 1 tsp. cinnamon powder
- ¼ c. cacao power
- 1 tsp. vanilla extract

Blend everything together in a food processor or blender until creamy.

Brownie Bites

- 1 c. raw walnut pieces
- 2 tbsp. raw cacao powder
- 1 tsp. salt
- 2 tbsp. peanut butter powder (optional)
- 1 tsp. vanilla extract

Grind all ingredients in a foods processor; roll out brownie bites using 1 tbsp. of the dough, and chill in the refrigerator.

Chocolate Dipped Strawberries

- 1 package large organic strawberries
- ½ c. coconut oil
- ½ c. raw cacao powder
- 1/2 tsp. sea salt
- ½ c. monk fruit powder

Melt the coconut oil on low heat, add remaining ingredients combine well. Dip strawberries in chocolate sauce and set on wax paper. Repeat with all the strawberries. Drizzle remaining chocolate over the strawberries for a second coating. Chill in the refrigerator for 30 minutes.

Health Remedies

Morning Kidney Flush

The kidneys are one of our excretory organs, meaning they have the job of excreting a substance that helps to clean the body. In this case, the kidneys and urinary system work together to clean and balance the fluid system in the body. Lemon juice and lemon oil (from the rind) both help stimulate the kidneys (as well as colon), making it a great every morning drink.

- 1-2 c. room temperature water
- 2 drops lemon essential oil
- 1 whole lemon

Fill a mug with water, add the juice of lemon, toss the lemon in, and add 2 drops of lemon oil. Drink it all within 1 hour of waking.

Natural Mouth Rinse

- 1 c. water
- 1/2 tsp. baking soda
- 1 drop peppermint essential oil

Blend everything together and gargle with the mixture morning and night.

Burn Soother

- ¼ c. aloe vera juice
- 5 drops lavender essential oil

Mix and store in the refrigerator. Use 1 tsp. at a time on burns.
Scrape and Scratch Ointment

- 1/4 c. coconut oil, melted
- 5 drops melaleuca oil

Blend ingredients and store in the refrigerator. Use topically on minor scrapes and cuts to disinfect.

Home and Garden

Hand Sanitizing Spray

- 10 drops essential oil such as lavender, melaleuca, geranium, lemon, peppermint, rosemary, or eucalyptus

Mix with water in a small spray bottle. This can be used on hands or anything you want to disinfect, such as shopping carts.

CONCLUSION

I look back over the last 20 years of my life and realize how long it took me to really get all this down. I know for most people it is a lot to digest and a lot of habits to break and rebuild. It is my hope that by laying this all out in 6 basic steps of what to include, you will be hitting the major points on what I feel have the greatest impact on your health. There will always be room for improvement, and we will always be learning new things about the body, and chemistry and science that come together to offer us more way to improve on our health and live in this crazy world!

For now my suggestion to all my readers, students and friends is to make a big push for 6-8 weeks. Make a commitment to yourself to be open minded, to try new ways of living each day, to begin to let go of old habits that don't serve you and to embrace the new ones that bring value to your life. It takes about 90 days to create new habits, so the longer you push yourself, the more likely you are to slide into that new habit zone where all of this becomes a natural part of life and something you enjoy doing!

One of the ways to create longevity in yoru program is to get organized, and come up with a plan to follow, I call it creating your "Personal Wellness Plan". This is a great way to take everything you have learned, apply it where you need to into a structured format. I recommend incorporating 1 item from 1 step each day, so that every day you are doing something that continues to move your health down the path that you want. I have students fill out a simple piece of paper that they draw into a calendar, giving yourself 7 days in a week, and then 4 row to complete a plan for the month (adjusting days as needed). Going down the list of steps, choose 1 item from each step and write it in the box for each day. These can be small things such as Sunday is prep-cooking, Monday is dry brushing, Tuesday is tea making etc. The point is to have a daily reminder and task to complete. This is extremely helpful as a self-coaching tool! Once you fill out the plan for the month, take notes in a journal each day for how you feel, any adjustments you want to make etc. At the end of the month, evaluate yourself. How do you feel, what do you need to emphasize next, and use those notes to create the next month. This can continue on form many months taking baby step, to big steps to finally reach all of your health goals. You will probably learn new skills and tools and over the course of several months our wellness plan will change and evolve several times. This is a very good thing. Remember that it takes time to instill new habits, but that is the key to change. This was the theme in my 20 year journey to health, I know it can be for you as well. Enjoy the journey!

"Happiness is not a destination, it's a way of life!"
– Unknown

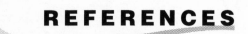

REFERENCES

Haeniein, George. "Lipids And Proteins In Milk, Particularly Goat Milk." *Lipids And Proteins In Milk, Particularly Goat Milk.* University of Delaware, n.d. Web. 03 June 2017.

Mayo Clinic. http://www.mayoclinic.org/diseases-conditions/inflammatory-bowel-disease/basics/definition/con-20034908

National Institutes of Health. https://www.ncbi.nlm.nih.gov/pmc/articles/PMC2290997/

National Institutes of Health, National Toxicology Program Report on Carcinogens (https://ntp.niehs.nih.gov/pubhealth/roc/index.html)

United States Enironmental Protection Agency https://www.epa.gov/radon/health-risk-radon

U.S. Food and Drug Administration. https://www.accessdata.fda.gov/scripts/cdrh/cfdocs/cfcfr/CFRSearch.cfm?fr=182.20

World Health Organization - www.who.int

Environmental Working Group www.EWG.org

GLOSSARY

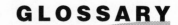

Adaptogen – a non-nutritional supplement which allegedly helps the body adapt to various stressors such as heat, cold, exertion, trauma, sleep deprivation, toxic exposure, radiation, infections and psychological stress.

Alkaline – having a pH greater than 7.

Antispasmodic – used o relieve spasm of involuntary muscle.

Astringent – causing the contraction of body tissues, typically of the skin. Used to protect the skin and assist with minor abrasions.

Autoimmune disease – a disease resulting from a disordered immune reaction in which antibodies are produced against ones' own tissues, as systemic lupus or rheumatoid arthritis.

Blood sugar – the concentration of glucose in the blood.

Carminative – relieves gas or flatulence.

Cortisol – a stress hormone made by the adrenal glands when the body is under stress. One of several steroid hormones produced by the adrenal cortex.

Diuretic – causing increased passing of urine

emmenagogue - stimulates the flow of menstrual bleeding.

Ghrelin – a hormone produced in the body that stimulates appetite.

Glucogon – a hormone secreted by the pancreas that acts in opposition to insulin in the regulation of blood glucose levels.

Glucose – a simple sugar that is an energy source in living organisms and is a component of many carbohydrates.

Glutathione – a compound involved as a coenzyme in oxidation-reduction reactions in cells.

Glycemic index – a value assigned to foods based on how slowly or how quickly those foods cause increases in blood sugar. A value of 100 represents the standard, an equivalent amount of pure glucose.

Glycogen – a polysaccharide deposited in bodily tissues as a store of carbohydrates.

Hepatic – stimulates the functions of the liver.

Insecticide – kills bugs and parasites.

Leptin – a satiety hormone produced by fatty tissue and believed to regulate fat storage in the body. Leptin may help regulate energy balance by inhibiting hunger.

Lymph – a colorless fluid containing white blood cells, which bathes the tissues and drains through the lymphatic system into the bloodstream.

Lymphatic System – the network of vessels through which lymph drains from the tissues into the blood.

Parabens – any group of compounds used as preservatives in pharmaceutical and cosmetic product sand in the food industry.

phthalates – a group of chemicals used to soften and increase flexibility of plastic materials. They are often found in vinyl, perfume, shampoo, nail polish and adhesives and are considered a possible carcinogen.

Pranayama – in Hindu yoga, the regulation of the breath through certain techniques and exercises.

Radon – a rare radioactive gas belonging to the noble gas series that is harmful to health.

Regenerative – tending to regenerate cells when used in the context of herbal medicine.

Rubefacient – a substance for topical application that produces redness of the skin causing dilation of the capillaries and an increase in blood circulation.

Sedative – increases sedation by reducing inability or excitement. In reference to herbal medicine refers to the calming affect on the body that may induce sleep.

Styptic – stops bleeding.

Tincture – a medicine made by dissolving a plant in alcohol.

Tonic – a medicinal substance taken to give a feeling of well-being.

Vasoconstrictor – the constriction of blood vessels, which increases blood pressure.

Vermifuge – an anthelmintic medicine that discourages parasites.

vulnerary - used in would healing

Xenoestrogen – a synthetic or natural chemical that imitates estrogen.

Printed in the United States
By Bookmasters